T0128751

Move On

Live Laugh Love Again

BERNICE S. DYSON

authorHOUSE®

AuthorHouse™
1663 Liberty Drive
Bloomington, IN 47403
www.authorhouse.com
Phone: 1-800-839-8640

© *2011 by Bernice S. Dyson. All rights reserved.*

No part of this book may be reproduced, stored in a retrieval system, or transmitted by any means without the written permission of the author.

First published by AuthorHouse   09/07/2011

ISBN: 978-1-4670-3322-0 (sc)
ISBN: 978-1-4670-3323-7 (ebk)

Library of Congress Control Number: 2011916268

Printed in the United States of America

Any people depicted in stock imagery provided by Thinkstock are models, and such images are being used for illustrative purposes only.
Certain stock imagery © Thinkstock.

This book is printed on acid-free paper.

Because of the dynamic nature of the Internet, any web addresses or links contained in this book may have changed since publication and may no longer be valid. The views expressed in this work are solely those of the author and do not necessarily reflect the views of the publisher, and the publisher hereby disclaims any responsibility for them.

CONTENTS

INTRODUCTION

"MOVE ON" HOW many times have you heard someone give this advice to someone else or even to you? These two words maybe two of the easiest words to say, but two of the most difficult words to do.

You've been through the fire that surely must feel like what we imagine hell to be like, way too many times than you care to remember. Now it's time to find a little touch of heaven here on earth.

There's no doubt it's waiting for you if you make it happen. You're going to have to move on and leave behind the nonsense, crap, abuse, bad relationships, bad jobs, liars, cheaters, and everything that's negative in your life to make it happen. It's not going to be easy because the reality is, life is like an obstacle course full of mental and physical challenges which are generally never easy, and this makes it a challenge. You're going to have to think and make your way through each and every challenge as they come.

The challenges will become easier no matter what they are once you make your mind up you can get through them. Everything starts with the mind then your body will follow its lead. Before you know it you will be exactly where you want to be and with whom you want to be with in this life.

There are millions of people around the world who have a story like mine, of a little girl growing up in Harlem who just wants to be happy,

1

and has dreams bigger than the city she lives in, but every time her dreams come to life there's yet another obstacle that's so overwhelming it either destroys her dreams or turns them into nightmares.

This little girl had to learn how to think, have courage and love herself enough to continuously move on in spite of the constant loss of loved ones, losing her two businesses, losing her house, all of her wealth, her mental health, bad and degrading relationships, poverty, and endless rollercoaster rides which would slowly take her to the top and quickly come down over and over again.

You too need to love yourself enough to know you deserve to be happy, live your life to the fullest, love and be loved. Starting today move on and make it happen.

ACKNOWLEDGEMENTS

- First and far most, I'd like to thank my lord and savior Jesus Christ. Without him nothing would be possible.
- Thank you to my lovely tweety bird. You've been there with me like no one else here on earth I will be forever grateful to you for loving me unconditionally. I love you more than life itself.
- To my friends that have been true friends and remained true friends, you will always be dear to me.
- To my family members that have had my back. I thank you and I love you
- To everyone that helped me in any small way with my first book. When I get the opportunity to thank you in some way, trust me I will, no matter how long it takes me. I love you and thank you from the bottom of my heart.

Sincerely, B.

CHAPTER 1

Moving On

I WAS TALKING WITH a friend about the problems she was having maintaining her house, she is a single mom working two jobs and couldn't seem to get a handle on all the bills that come with owning a house.

This particular day she was especially upset. My friend had just found out if your grass grows to high you can be fined, she couldn't afford to pay someone to cut her grass anymore therefore, she would have to start cutting it herself. I suggested she get someone to move in with her to help her with the expenses. My friend looked at me as her eyes started tearing up and told me she doesn't have anyone and she would rather kill herself than lose her house.

I told my friend not to say this and not to worry, everything will be okay. I'm sure she thought I was just trying to console her by saying everything will be okay, but the truth is I had been through the very pain that she was so afraid to face and I knew for a fact it would be okay.

Throughout the past seven years not only did I lose my house but I lost my husband, my six figure salary, my businesses, my car, all my wealth and my mind. I've been in several self-destructive romantic relationships, lived in apartments that were dumps, and worked numerous close to minimum wage jobs. These years were like a slow painful death. I didn't try to kill myself, I had to find the strength and courage to move on from some of the most devastating and challenging obstacles a person has to move on from.

It is not easy which is why it's a challenge, but if you can think properly, dream, have courage, and love yourself you can move on from anything.

On my journey to reconstruct my life after so much destruction I realized I needed help to gain back all the qualities I had that allowed me to progress in the first place. I started seeing a therapist, she helped me to reconstruct my way of thinking which helped me to get my mind right. Your mind controls everything you do including self-destructive behavior.

In my case I was suffering from a mental illness called depression. My illness stripped me of my courage, ability to make good decisions, strength, self-love, and self-esteem. Once I was able to re-gain these most important qualities back they became instrumental factors in my recovery. I had to take all my negative thoughts and turn them into positive thoughts. Instead of thinking I can't or I'm not, I had to think I can and I will, for instance, I had to start thinking I can do a particular thing because I am not afraid instead of thinking I can't do something because I am afraid. I had to stop thinking I'm not going to be able to fulfill my dreams and start thinking I am going to be able to fulfill my dreams.

Everyone's situation is different, but no matter what your situation is, obstacle or crisis is, you're going to have to be capable of thinking positively, have courage, love yourself, be strong, have standards, and not be afraid to dream then you will be able to get through anything.

One of the first moves I've ever made that required a substantial amount of courage happened a little over ten years ago when my daughter was in pre-school. As I was picking up my daughter from school I noticed her little head was lying on the desk while the other children were on their mats taking a nap. I asked one of the staff members why wasn't my daughter laying down? She told me her blanket wasn't clean. I started yelling so loud that I woke up every child in the place. I told this staff member and everyone else that was listening I had just bought my daughters blanket the day before and I just heard the most stupid excuse I've ever heard in my life. I then said I had better take my daughter and go before someone gets hurt. My daughter and I left and never returned.

I was now faced with the obstacle of not having childcare so I started looking for other pre-schools but didn't find any I approved of. My family was helping by watching my daughter as I was looking for a new pre-school, but they had jobs of their own so I did what I had to do and quit my job.

At this time in my life my mind was sharp. I was brought up in a home where dreams come true so I knew how to dream. I understood how important it is to have courage to progress in life and make your dreams come true, otherwise you'll be crippled by fear and unable to move on. I loved my daughter and I loved myself. I had all the ingredients I needed to move on with my life, with or without a job so that's exactly what I did.

I thought of a plan to ensure I could work and my daughter would have childcare. I took a few classes at a local college for six weeks on how to start a daycare center I registered my new business and passed out some flyers in the neighborhood. Before long I had started my first business, had a job and no longer had the obstacle of not having child care for my daughter.

Possessing the following qualities will enable you to do anything that you want to do. What the mind can conceive the body can achieve.

- Be capable of thinking properly
- Have courage, face your fears. Don't be afraid to meet the challenge of obstacles. This is the only way you will make it through your journey in life. Life is full of obstacles you cannot avoid them
- Love yourself enough to know you deserve to live the best quality of life possible. You deserve to be happy and laugh. You deserve to love someone whose worthy of your love and who loves you the way you deserve to be loved.
- Don't be too proud to seek help when you need it, even therapist go to therapist for help.
- Learn how to let go of unhealthy relationships and be forgiving. You will never be capable of moving into the future if you can't forgive and let go of the past.
- Try to always have a plan of action. Your life will flow much easier if you plan out where you would like to go and what you would like to do.

The most important thing you will have to do if you're in a position of needing to move on is making sure you're in the right state of mind. To do so if your depressed, doubting yourself, not loving yourself or having a great deal of negative thoughts about your abilities, you probably won't be able to move on successfully, until you can turn your frame of mind around. This is a perfect time to get help. You can either go to a therapist, a family member, a friend, a church member, a school counselor, or a social worker and ask for help. You will need to think positively and clearly in order for you to make a good move that's going to benefit you and ultimately bring you happiness.

I expanded my childcare business and started another business B.S.D entertainment, an entertainment management company.

Both of my businesses were doing extremely well and my husband was doing well with his career so we decided to buy our first house and do a little traveling. I was on top of the world with my head in the clouds.

I felt like I could fly, until the unthinkable happened, my husband became ill, had a heart attack and passed away. I was like a plane that was just in the sky flying over the clouds that came down to a crash landing. I remember thinking this couldn't be happening, but it was and it was just a preview of what was to come.

When my husband passed away, not only did I lose my husband but I lost my mind. I was in trouble and my mind wasn't right enough for me to realize I needed help. I can't emphasize enough when your mind isn't right you won't have any form of reasonable or rational thinking, so you won't be able to overcome the numerous obstacles you'll face in your life in order to move on, progress and be happy.

The obstacles will control you and you'll be completely lost and start to regress. Like anyone who loses their mind, I started losing control of my life. I lost the first business I started, safe care childcare which was paying me a six figure salary. Shortly after that I lost the second business I started B.S.D entertainment that was adding a substantial amount of income to my salary.

I then lost my beautiful split level four bedroom, three bathroom house on the Southside of Freeport, New York which included a pool, an enormous backyard with a fully furnished deck. Inside my house was even more fabulous. I had leather furnishings, oriental rugs and tiffany ceiling fixtures. My finished basement had wall to wall mirrors, surrounding a fully stocked bar with a laundry room right around the corner. I always hated going to the Laundromat, so having a laundry room was a dream in its self. Close your eyes and vision a beautiful house by the water. This is what I lost. If this wasn't enough I then lost my car.

Once I was finally able to think well enough to realize I needed help I became humble and sought professional help. I started psychotherapy, and other related treatments which focused on me getting my mind and body functioning positively again. It took sometime but gradually I was able to start making rational decisions again.

I started getting back my strength and my ability to think about the goals and dreams that I wanted to achieve. I started having control over my life and planning once again for my future. Once I became mentally stronger, I started dealing with the obstacles that are designed to hold you back from progressing in a different manner. I started moving on from, and making moves to get away from some of the bad situations I have gotten into when my mind wasn't functioning properly

I had lived in a basement apartment that wasn't up to anyone's standard of living, and had shared an apartment with a lady that was crazier than I was. I moved on from these situations and got my own apartment. I was working jobs that was paying as low as nine dollars and change an hour. I went back to school so I could stop working practically for free and be able to improve my quality of life.

I was involved in six bad romantic relationships in which I was lied to, played, and disrespected in ways I didn't even know were possible. Since therapy I've been able to fully move on by exercising the standards, self-love and respect I have for myself. Last but not least I regained my courage and dared to dream again.

Obstacles will always exist their challenging mental and physical tests, which is why you have to be mentally fit. If you're not mentally fit you won't be physically fit and able to endure your many challenges. Our entire journey in life is like an obstacle course. Once you get pass one obstacle another one shows up from nowhere. Some of these obstacles will knock you to your knees. Say a little prayer then get back up and keep moving. Never say never, Always say in due time. With your mind right you can move on and progress from anything. Take it a day at a time take it slow, but never stay still if a situation is a problem, you must resolve it. Problems never just resolve themselves. If a problem becomes a load too heavy for you to carry drop the load and move on or you'll be sure to sink.

Move on towards your dreams

As you move on, you want to move on to bigger and better things. You want to pursue your dreams and goals. You want to aspire to make your life the best it can be. In order for you to make great things happen in your life, you need to have a vision or a dream of what it is you want. There aren't any dreams that are out of your reach, you have to dare to reach them. You can reach for the stars if you want to. If you want to move on to a dream job, you can. If you have the desire to purchase a dream house, you can. If you want to have a wonderful relationship, with a fabulous man of your dreams, then that's what you pursue.

Once you have the courage and dare to dream you can make any dream come true. Don't just move on; move on toward your dreams of greatness.

When I was a kid growing up in Harlem, I use to look out my eleventh floor window and day dream about how my life was going to be when I grew up. Dreaming was something that I was taught in my home.

My parents had a picture of Dr. Martin Luther king Jr. over their bed on a plaque next to his I have a dream speech. My siblings and I were taught it's important to have dreams and they can come true, but you have to make them happen. My mother always told us to be humble and ask for god's help, but god helps those that help themselves, so you have to help yourself first.

My mother also told us not to be afraid of working hard for what you want in this life. Nothing in life is easy, but with hard work and perseverance, you can do anything you want to do as long as you don't let anything or anyone get in your way. My mother talked the talk and walked the walk.

As a youth I looked, listened, and learned as my mother turned her dreams into realities. Mom was a nursing assistant with dreams of becoming a doctor. I watched her first become a licensed practical nurse at a local community center nursing program. She then became a registered nurse. She later received her master degree in nursing from Columbia University then enrolled in medical school.

What a lesson I learned over these years about dreams, courage, strength, and determination. My mother showed me what she had talked about all along, through her actions. There was a dream, a plan of action, and the courage to move past all the obstacles that were presented in order to make that dream a reality.

There were many obstacles and they weren't few and in-between. When it rained it poured. However my mother being as mentally strong as she is, the obstacles may have slowed her down a little but they didn't stop her.

My father was a good father, but he wasn't a good husband to my mother. My mom and dad fought often about her going to school. My father became a big obstacle in the way of my mother's success. Eventually they separated. I was heartbroken, but not surprised. I knew my mother was a firm believer in not letting obstacles get in the way, and stop you from accomplishing your dreams, unfortunately this included an unsupportive spouse.

The obstacles continued to plague my mother. My grandmother became ill, so my mother had to care for her while she attended medical school. While caring for my grandmother, my mother became ill as well and had to leave medical school. She was down for the count but not out. Once she got back on her feet she worked as a nurse, bought herself a beautiful two family house, a new car, traveled and provided a better quality of life for herself and her family.

My mother becoming ill taught me another very important lesson. Some obstacles are so tough they will knock you out like in a heavy weight fight, but you have to get back up and keep fighting until you become victorious and achieve your goals.

If you're going to be truly happy, you will probably have to move on from negative situations many times in your lifetime. Sometimes your move will be a choice, other times it will be a necessity, but there will always be an obstacle involved. You will never be able to move on if you can't get past the obstacles.

Every obstacle is either mentally challenging, physically challenging, or both. You will need to be mentally and physically fit in order to defeat your challenges. You have to know and believe that you are that fierce person that dreams, faces their fears, knows how to love, especially yourself, gives and demands respect, knows what you want and how to plan for it, and isn't to proud to be humble.

CHAPTER 2

Get your mind right

YOUR MIND IS the commander of your body. If your mind tells your body to be strong it will. The mind is so powerful, that if your mind is weak and all you have left is your body, the first bit of pain your body feels it will not be able to fight without the strength of your mind telling it to fight. Your body will not be able to fight.

Train your mind to make decisions your body will obey. As your reading this book, tell your mind to lift your right arm. You will lift your right arm. I've gone to day classes, night classes, and weekend classes. Each semester that I've had a class that wasn't a traditional Monday through Friday class that met in the daytime, I had to tell my mind you have to go to class in order for my body to obey.

When obstacles and crisis would arise, my mind would tell my body to meet the challenge. My mind would meet the mental challenge and my body would meet the physical challenge. It was never easy, because life isn't easy but that's why it is a challenge. Just remember what the mind can conceive the body can achieve.

If you find yourself in a situation that your wondering how you're going to get through it, tell yourself you can do it, convince yourself you can get through anything then you will be able to take the appropriate steps to do so. We do this all the time. We make it through that day we could barely drag ourselves out of bed. We finish that project we never thought we would finish, or we've made it pass that bad situation we had to move on from six months ago and we are still standing on our feet.

No matter how the following may sound it will prove to be true. Challenge yourself and try the following. Tell your mind you can do something that maybe a little challenging for you. Continue to tell yourself over and over again, convince yourself that you can do it, then attempt to do it. You will see you can and will do what you are attempting to do.

Start off with something small, then gradually increase the degree of difficulty of your challenge. For instance try a new project you always wanted to do or try going somewhere by yourself that you would never go, like a restaurant or a movie theater. Gradually try something more challenging like giving up a bad habit of drinking every day and try to limit your drinking to social drinking.

With each challenge that you meet you will see you can do whatever you set your mind to do. You'll begin to feel more confident at attempting those bigger challenges end life, like moving on from bad relationships, dead in jobs, or any negative situation that exist in your life.

One experience everyone has gone through is taking a new class. This is usually always challenging. You had to learn new material you did not know, until you were able to complete the course. Each new job you started was a new challenge. Once you learned how to do what was required of you, your challenge was met. We've had to learn new challenges since we learned how to talk, walk, and eat. When I started my businesses, I could barely keep a balanced checkbook. Running and operating an entire business was a huge challenge.

I started learning through self-help books, education and experience. As time went on I gained the knowledge I needed and became very successful at what I was doing.

Knowledge

Knowledge is the result of perception, learning, and reasoning. You gain expertise and skills through experience, education, the practical understanding of a subject and time.

Have you ever heard someone sing, play an instrument, or lecture a class that was so good all you could say was wow, that person has skills. Well that person has knowledge of what they are doing, probably gained by a combination of experience, education, and an understanding of the subject matter which resulted in them doing it so well.

The more knowledge you have about something, the more successful you'll be at it. Feed your mind knowledge or it will slowly waste away. The mind is a terrible thing to waste. Gain knowledge about everything that's going on in your life and the world around you. The more you know, the wiser your decisions will be that you make. You won't ever be capable of making an educated decision about something or someone you don't know anything about.

Knowledge through Books

You can gain a world of knowledge from a book. Whatever your obstacle is, whatever you need to know, you can learn about it in a book. I've learned a great deal about cooking, decorating, relationships, personalities, starting a business, and many other subject matters all from books.

Schools use books as a primary learning tool for teaching. The authors who write these books are sharing their personal expertise, things they have experienced and learned with you to enlighten you of the knowledge they have. Take advantage of it. Let's say you were going to Spain to live, where Spanish is the primary language spoken. It may be a good idea to read a book or go to a class where a textbook would be used and learn a little Spanish before you go to Spain to live.

In my opinion the greatest book ever written is the bible. How many times throughout our lives have we gotten a scripture out of the bible to help us get through some crisis. Gaining knowledge from books is so relevant, that one of the most trained professionals, doctors have used books as one of their primary learning tools for years. Go inside any doctor's office and look at the wall right next to their degrees on the bookshelf, you will find dozens of books that they've read and got knowledge from for years.

Lawyers refer to books for each case they represent. You may hear a lawyer commonly say something like, in the case of harry vs. harry, their referring to a case they've gotten out of a book that's very similar to their present case.

Utilize books as another source of information that can help you move on from an obstacle that you will face as you attempt to progress on your journey.

Experience

One of the best ways to gain knowledge is through experience. Learn from your past experiences and mistakes as well as the achievements you have made and goals you have reached. Let the negative experiences in your life become an example of what you shouldn't do, like sleeping with someone before getting a chance to know them, because they may disappear, or driving drunk and nearly killing yourself.

Let the positive things you've experienced be an example for how you should live your life, like making a move from a bad situation which resulted in your life being much happier and healthier. Knowing you can start a business and make it successful or move on to another job, and be successful at it will give you the positive reinforcement you need to do it again without fear.

My personal experience is the knowledge I'm using to share with you. I've studied people and their personalities for years, but nothing has been able to enrich my life more than the experiences I've had in my life. My experiences provided me with real life learning vs. the theories that I've learned from textbooks. Don't get me wrong, theories are very helpful, because their someone else's experiences, but there's no better experience then your own.

Meditation

Meditation is silencing the mind. By silencing your mind you will be able to clear away the distractions that interfere with thinking clearly. It is vitally important to think clearly when faced with an obstacle or challenge that requires you to move on. Meditation works on strengthening the mind by training or re-programing your way of thinking.

Meditation relaxes your mind and conditions your mind to better control emotional anxiety. This is very important, because moving on from something or someone who was once a comfort zone for you can be very upsetting and cause anxiousness or anxiety. Meditation also encourages self-love, improving our relationship with ourselves, and high self-esteem.

Act of Meditation

- Try to meditate every day.
- Find a place and time you won't be disturbed.
- Don't eat before meditating (you'll be so relaxed you might fall asleep)
- Sit with a straight back.
- Find a focal point (a candle flame is one suggestion).
- Concentrate on your focal point, on that one item, block out all other thoughts.
- Once you learn how to concentrate on one thing, your next step will be no thoughts at all.

Meditation is one of those mental challenges that is very difficult, but like every challenge with practice, experience, and over time it becomes easier to reject thoughts into your mind. You will want to have a clear mind and experience inner peace in the mist of conquering all the challenges that may come your way.

Exercise

Before taking on any exercise routine, it is strongly recommended to check with a health care professional as to what level of exercise is appropriate for you. Once you have consulted with a physician, start a fitness routine.

Anyone who has gone to a gym will be able to tell you, one of the most challenging things about having a regular fitness routine is finding the time to go to the gym. To insure that your routine is one that you can stick to, design a routine that will fit your schedule. Set your own pace. Start slow and gradually progress.

There are so many different types of exercise you can include into your fitness routine. Most of them will strengthen your body for those physical challenges. They will also reduce your risk of diseases, help you lose weight, improve coordination and balance, improve your sleeping habits, and help you look even better which will improve your self-esteem.

I've checked with some trainers at the gym. This is a list of some of the most recommended exercises you can do and a little bit about what they will do for you.

- Weight training—strengthens and improves your muscles.
- Pushups—works your chest, triceps, back, and abs.
- The plank (used in Pilates)—works the back, abs, arms, legs, and internal abdominal muscles.
- Lunges—work most of the muscles in your legs, including your quads, hamstrings, gluts, and calves.

- Aerobics—dance routines that work the entire body.
- Squats—work your gluts, hamstrings, quads, and calves.
- Lat pull-down—strengthens your back and helps to burn calories.
- Yoga and stretching—stress reduction, spiritual growth, helps with sleep disorders, allergy and asthma symptom relief, lower heart rate, lower blood pressure, increased strength and flexibility, improvement of many medical conditions, reduces anxiety, reduces muscle tension, reduces cortisol levels, and slows the aging process.

Diet

I am sure you've heard the saying you are what you eat. What you eat influences along with exercise how you look and how you feel. One of the obstacles in everyone's life is trying to eat a good balanced diet in order to be as healthy as possible. A balanced diet will provide your body with energy and nutrition for the healthy growth and development of your body and mind.

Choose a wide variety of foods and drinks from all of the food groups. Eat and drink in moderation. Too much of anything is not good for you. Use moderation especially when in taking saturated fat, Trans fat cholesterol, refined sugar, salt, and alcohol. Be considerate of calorie levels and portion control.

This is a guide of the major food groups and the foods included in these groups. Always try to eat at least three meals a day, never skip breakfast and remember moderation and portion control are key.

Fruit groups

- Apples
- Apricots
- Avocadoes
- Bananas
- Berries
- Dates
- Grapes
- Grapefruit
- Tangerines
- Oranges
- Unsweetened dried fruit
- Raisins
- Pineapples
- Peaches
- Melons
- Mangos
- 100% fruit juices

Vegetable groups

- Tomatoes
- Sweet potatoes
- Squash
- Broccoli
- Carrots
- Cauliflower
- Collard greens
- Cucumbers
- Green beans
- Spinach
- Kale
- Potatoes
- Lettuce
- Radishes
- 100% vegetable juices

Dairy

- Yogurt—fat free or low fat
- Milk or buttermilk—fat free skim milk or 1% low fat
- Cheese—fat free or reduced fat

Lean animal proteins

- Meat—beef, pork, poultry with the skin removed, game meats, meats should be broiled, poached or roasted.

Fish

- Most types of fish, shell fish in particular.

Beans

- Lentils
- Peas
- Split peas
- Most beans

Nuts and seeds

- Walnuts
- Almonds
- Sunflower
- Peanuts
- Peanut butter
- Seeds
- Hazel nuts
- Mixed nuts

Unsaturated fats

- Olive oil
- Vegetable oil\
- Low fat mayonnaise
- Light or low-fat salad dressing

Soy milk

Soy milk will provide protein which affects brain performance. The protein provides amino acids from which neurotransmitters are made of. Neurotransmitters carry signals from one brain cell to another. The more you feed these messengers, the more efficient they are.

Cacao beans

This is one healthy food you'll find in most dark chocolate bars and cacao. If you mix 100% organic cacao powder with espresso, organic unsweetened soy milk, cinnamon, and a sprinkle of cayenne red pepper it will make a brain and body stimulating drink.

Green tea

Green tea powder that you will find in green tea contains epigallocatechin gallate, an anti-cancer and anti-aging compound found uniquely in green tea. Green tea powder also helps you to become calm, focused and stimulated at the same time.

CHAPTER 3

Courage

Fear can sometimes take over all rational thoughts. Fear can cause you to panic, be afraid, anxious or apprehensive about a possible or probable situation. Your fear may be based on a real situation. If someone or something hurts you, you may have a reason to fear it in the future. Your fear may be based on a possible situation like, what could possibly happen if you move on.

Fear may cause you to avoid a possible threat. Your fear may be based on an exaggerated situation. You may recall past similar fears or occurrences and inject them into your current situation.

Courage is being able to face these fears. Courage is the primary driver of any action. If we lose our courage, our ability to act in the face of a risk, we'll never be able to achieve anything.

Not facing your fears can cripple you. You'll be paralyzed and not able to progress and move onto the next level in your life, where your goals and dreams can come to life once you make it through the necessary journey.

The unknown

We often worry what could possibly happen if we move on? The unknown can be very frightening. Fear is an emotional obstacle that is an instinctual response to a potential danger, or a possibility of what could happen. When you move on, most of your fears could derive from the unknown questions like, suppose this happens or what if that happens?

Most people are afraid of taking risks. Every time you move on, there is a risk of how the outcome will turn out. To get rid of the fear derived from the uncertainty of a situation, have a plan.

Prepare yourself with a plan A and a plan B. Consider every possible outcome and how you can handle each outcome. For instance if you plan on moving on from an abusive relationship, this may leave you without a home and money, plan accordingly.

Try to find a new place to live and get a job before moving from your present situation. Remember most fears derive from probable or possible situations or outcomes. If you prepare yourself for these outcomes, you'll have nothing to fear but fear itself. It's not going to be easy, but then that's why it's an obstacle, physically and mentally challenging. Also remember nothing in life is for certain except death.

Comfort zone

Everyone has a comfort zone, things and people that they are comfortable with. These comfort zones are safety barriers we surround ourselves with to protect us from feelings of hurt. If we could learn to step out of our comfort zones, this could help us with dealing with the unknown. Try some of the following things to help you to feel comfortable outside of your comfort zone.

- Do something you wouldn't ordinarily do (start off small)
- Don't always hesitate when trying something new, for instance when we learn how to swim; we should just jump in without worrying how cold the water will be. It may be cold initially, but your body will adjust.

Root of your fear

Fear can be derived from an experience you've had that was bad and you never faced it head on to get rid of the fear. Is the origin of the fear something that has a probability of being a regular occurrence, or is it more of a delusional or distorted way of looking at things?

When I was eleven years old my mother's friend's husband was pushed in front of a moving train on Christmas day. I was afraid of trains for years after this occurred.

When I was a teenager and old enough to travel on my own I took a bus to get where ever I had to go. If a bus couldn't get me there I wouldn't go. I started driving when I was 20 years old, and have been driving since. I thought I was safe from ever being faced with having to take a train again, until my license was suspended for unpaid tickets. I still was afraid of taking trains, since I was driving most of the time I didn't have to take trains often, so I never faced my fear of trains.

While I was working on getting my license situation straightened out I still needed to get around. I tried taking a bus to get everywhere I needed to get to, but with the busy schedule I had, there just weren't enough hours in the day for me to get to places on time.

I was faced with the dilemma of either losing my job and flunking out of school, or taking a train. I decided I wasn't going to let my fear of trains stop me from moving on and progressing with my life. For three weeks straight I took a train to where I had to go.

At first I would stand by the stairs until the train came to a complete stop then run onto the train. After about four days, I actually stood on the platform, but against the wall until the train came to a complete stop, then I would run on the train. In about a week I was no longer holding onto the wall and felt comfortable at the mid-way point between the wall and the tracks. After riding on trains for three weeks I could actually look at the train as it was coming into the station. I never stood at the edge of the tracks, because I am no fool, but I was no longer afraid of getting on the train.

I faced my fear, so now I have one less situation in my life that causes me anxiety or cripples me from achieving my dreams.

Unbelievable courage

I'm sure we've all had stories like mine of being afraid of one thing or another. If not trains then planes or getting on a bicycle for the very first time. Once we've done it repeatedly and faced our fear, we are no longer afraid. This is courage. Facing those fears until we no longer have the fear.

I've seen some acts of courage that would make getting on an air plane, moving on from an abusive relationship or handing in a resignation look like a walk in the park. These people had the courage to die.

I used to work in a hospital in the hospice unit for four years. A hospice unit is a unit in the hospital that you go to for palliative care as your dying. There's nothing more courageous than facing death with dignity.

Joseph

Joseph was a 28 year old Jamaican man, who came to hospice diagnosed with cancer. He was a very handsome, soft spoken man. He was a fifth grade school teacher. When Joseph first walked onto the hospice unit, I was surprised at how well he looked. His skin was so beautiful. His complexion was so clear. His facial hair was well groomed and his body looked fit. He did not look sick at all.

As I was getting Joseph settled into hospice I got to know him a little. He always wanted to teach and loved his children in his fifth grade class that he taught. He talked about each and every one of his students by name and their distinctive personalities.

I checked on Joseph many times throughout my shift and he very seldom needed anything or wanted anything outside of his medication for the excruciating pain he must have been in. Joseph remained this way for the first two and a half weeks he was on hospice.

Toward the end of Josephs third week on hospice his vitals started declining. Joseph finally had a request. In his normal soft spoken voice, Joseph asked to see his brother who was in prison. We took josephs request to administration. It took some doing, but we were able to get josephs request granted.

It was a Sunday afternoon when Josephs brother was escorted to the hospice unit in shackles. After taking one look at Joseph, this 6foot something 300 pound man dressed from head to toe in prison fatigue started crying. There wasn't a dry eye on the unit except Joseph. Joseph kept telling his brother, it's alright; it's going to be alright.

Joseph died the next day. Everyone on the hospice unit said to each other, Joseph must have been waiting for his brother to come so he could see him one more time to say goodbye.

Lisette

Lisette was a 26 year old Latin American female with two small children, ages three and five. Lisette came to hospice with cancer. When Lisette first stepped on the hospice unit she came with an entourage of about twelve people. We were touched, she had so many people showing her support, but at the same time this is a small six bed hospice unit where keeping our patients comfortable was our first priority.

We were concerned that so many people would generate a lot of noise, which could be a problem. Unlike what we thought, all of Lisette's support proved to be very helpful to her. The noise that came from her room wasn't the noise we was expecting at all. The noise from Lisette's room was the sounds of crying. Not Lisette crying, but the crying of her family and friends.

We never saw Lisette cry, but we often saw Lisette comforting her husband, mother, children, family, and friends. Lisette showed so much strength and courage. She smiled at times and was gracious at other times. There was so much family and friends around, Lisette seldom needed our assistance for anything except to give her, her medication.

One day Lisette called me in her room and asked me "can I ask you to do me a favor" this kind of caught me off guard because she very seldom called us to do anything for her, I said sure anything, what can I do for you? She said "I love the fragrance you're wearing, can you get me some, so I can smell good for my husband? I don't have much time left I'd love for him to remember me smelling good" I told Lisette sure I'll see what I can do, I'll be right back.

I knew we wasn't supposed to accept or give gifts to the patients, this was one of the hospitals rules, but I asked my supervisor if I could get Lisette some of the perfume I was wearing so she could put it on for her husband. My supervisor said yes.

I went back to Lisette's room and told her I would bring her some perfume the next day. She told me "thank you I'll put you in my prayers." Lisette died four days later. I'm so glad I gave her the fragrance and she gave me a lesson on courage. Lisette was courageous and gracious until the day she died.

CHAPTER 4

Love Yourself

WHEN I WAS a kid, like a lot of kids, there were so many things about myself that I either disliked or hated.

I use to think I was too tall and thin because I was 5'6 and slender when most of my friends were short, 5'3 and chubbier.

I had a head full of hair, that I didn't know how to style, I always thought my teeth were too big for my mouth.

I tried to gain weight, did so many different things to my hair until at one point it started to fall out and I tried not to smile.

It took me a long time to realize these were flaws I believed I had and everyone had their own flaws because no one is perfect.

I even learned to love my flaws. I realized it wasn't so bad being tall and thin with a head full of hair and a mouth full of teeth.

Since I've become an adult, I've developed a whole new set of flaws and have learned to love them all.

This is how you love yourself.

In spite of the flaws, through the good days, the bad days and the in between days, you still love yourself for who you are.

Taking care of yourself when you wake up in the morning, showering, brushing your teeth, fixing your hair, ironing your clothes, making sure your appearance is neat and getting a little something healthy to eat is loving yourself.

Ensuring you get and do the things necessary for yourself to have a good quality of life like a healthy immune boosting diet which promotes good health an exercise of your choice and some level of mental stimulation is loving yourself.

Once your basic needs for survival are met you're going to have other needs that will be important to your happiness.

We all have a need to pursue our dreams and goals, belong to someone or something, feel needed, special, loved, appreciated and respected.

Dreams and goals though we share with others are personal.

Only you can dream your dreams, have goals and make them come true.

Only you can believe in yourself enough to know that you can succeed at whatever you attempt to do.

No one will believe you are special or appreciate you if you don't believe you are special and appreciate yourself.

Love and respect is usually reciprocated.

The love and respect you will want and need someone to give you, you will need to know how to give it as well.

You will never be able to truly love anybody else if you don't love yourself first.

If this were a perfect world the people we love would love us back, but often this doesn't happen because this is an imperfect world.

Your need for love will never be met by someone who isn't loving you back, therefore you should move on until you find someone who loves you the way you need to be loved and deserve to be loved. Love yourself enough to understand and appreciate all the wonderful qualities you have that are worthy of loving.

Respect is also reciprocated, and earned.

Love yourself enough to respect yourself then you will earn the respect of others.

Have standards that say I respect my mind, my body and my soul and others will as well.

Physiological Needs

Since we were born we needed the basic things like food, air, sleep and water to survive.

When we were a few months old our parents took us to get the necessary immunizations so our bodies could fight off all those diseases that could affect our survival like measles, mumps and rubella.

As we continue to get older, the need for air, food, sleep, water and our bodies being able to fight off diseases will always be the most important basic needs we will ever have for the duration of our lives.

Drink plenty of water your body is made up of fifty to seventy five percent water, you can't live without it.

Get plenty of sleep, while your sleeping your body heals itself.

Get as much fresh air as possible, Protect yourself from the sun by using sunscreen daily, but ensure you get a little sun it's a wonderful source of vitamin D.

Eat foods that support your immune system. They will help keep you healthy and disease free.

The following are some immune boosting healthy diet foods:

- Kale is a vegetable that is a rich source of beta carotene which fights off colds and the flu. Your liver converts beta carotene into vitamin A. This vitamin builds up the immune system by increasing the production of whole blood cells. Vitamin A also helps maintain the lining of the respiratory and digestive tracts which are your first lines of defense against pathogens.

- Oats like you'll find in oatmeal are an excellent source of zinc, which builds your immunity. Oats also contain beta-glucan, a compound which activates immune cells that fight infectious microorganisms.
- Milk is fortified with vitamin D activates T cells, the immune systems virus-killing cells.
- Strawberries are very high in vitamin C. This vitamin reduces the severity of symptoms associated with the cold and flu. Vitamin C is also essential for maintaining healthy skin which is the bodies' first defense against viruses.
- Beans are full of vitamin B, which produces new immune cells. Beans are also high in soluble fiber which increases the production of an anti-inflammatory protein that strengthens the immune system.
- Green Tea leaves stimulate immune cells and fight the influenza virus.

One of the most deadly pandemics we've had as a nation in a long times is acquired immune deficiency syndrome or AIDS.

Aids is a disease of the human immune system cause by the human immunodeficiency Virus (HIV).

Over thirty three million people are living with the AIDS Virus.

Over two million new cases of AIDS are reported every year, that's not to mention the cases that are not reported.

Over a million AIDS related deaths occur per year.

Aids progressively reduce the effectiveness of the immune system and leaves individuals susceptible to infections.

Aids is transmitted through direct contact of a mucous membrane or the bloodstream with a bodily fluid containing HIV, such as blood semen, vaginal fluid, preseminal fluid and breast milk.

Aids is most commonly transmitted through sex, anal, vaginal or oral.

Love yourself enough to protect yourself. Do not have unprotected sex.

There is no known cure for HIV or Aids.

The nation is trying to keep this pandemic under control by emphasizing prevention.

Safe sex is the number one prevention for HIV and Aids, so always use a condom.

Safety Needs

Everyone has the need to feel safe. Often these needs for safety are threatened or compromised in some way like in an abusive home environment, marriage, school or even a job.

Many times people compromise themselves and stay in homes, marriages, jobs or schools for a false sense of security or because they believe they have no other available choices at the time.

There isn't any security if you're not safe. There's always another option to any situation. You simply may need help in figuring out what these options are.

Thousands of people are abused or killed in their own homes by significant others per year. Thousands of people are sexually harassed or abused at their jobs by their superiors and thousands more are bullied in their schools every year.

Have a plan of action to get away from these situations ASAP (As soon as possible).

If you feel lost or confused and don't know what to do go to a family member, friend, church member or counselor for help immediately.

If you can't get the help you need from any of these sources call the National Domestic Violence hotline at 1-800-799-Safe or the Abuse Victim Hotline at 877-448-8678.

Esteem Needs

In a world where there are so many various obstacles we have to get through, chaos we have to face, and people who are marching through life to the beat of their own drum, we have a need for law and order.

Everyone has to live by these laws every day, which are rules and regulations, or they'll have to pay the consequence.

If you kill someone you're breaking the law and will have to pay a consequence.

If you rape someone you're breaking the law and will have to pay a consequence. If you rob a bank, you're breaking the law and will have to pay a consequence.

Usually the consequence for breaking these laws or rules is incarceration or worse.

The people who break these laws are sociopaths and are alienated from the very society they are committing these crimes against.

No one should be exposed to people that would do these horrific things.

Your life should be operated in the same manner.

You should love yourself enough that you set standards for how you want to be treated by people.

You should have rules and guidelines that govern what you consider to be acceptable behavior and treatment from other people. If these rules are not followed there should be consequences.

Try to ensure that the consequence will not be something that will come back to haunt you. Alienation from that person will be the best choice for you to make as a repayment for being mistreated.

Remember you're the good person who knows how to give love; respect and appreciation, alienation from you will be an appropriate punishment. When you move on it will be their loss.

Don't seek revenge by any form of violence or wrong doings. What goes around comes around. Eventually you will be the one who will have a consequence to pay. If this is, or was your form of thinking when put in a situation in which you were mistreated, move on past this kind of negative thinking. Think positively even good things can come out of some bad situations. The sooner you get away from evil the better you will be.

Growing up if someone messed with me I had at least a dozen people I could go to that would handle the situation for me. The results were never very pretty.

This is not the way to live your life because you have to answer to god and his punishments are much worse than anything you, or any of your people will do to anybody else, because the punishments will be given to you and why should you be made to suffer further for someone else's evil actions when you've suffered enough already.

Do yourself a huge favor and just move on.

I started learning about having standards for myself when I was about twelve years old.

I am the youngest of four children so my brothers and sisters always had to look after me and my siblings were very close, partly because my mother was a single mother working two jobs and going to school so we took care of each other.

My oldest brother loved the girls and they loved him.

I noticed he would bring one around the block but never the apartment, then she would disappear after a few weeks.

Then a new one would start coming around for a few weeks then she would disappear.

Often times there would be different girls coming around at different times of the day all looking for my brother.

Sometimes they would come around the block at the same time and bump into each other; my brother wouldn't even blink an eye. It was as though he didn't care if they knew about each other.

Some of them even knew each other.

A lot of times these girls would just sit in the park with my brother and be fondled then they would go into one of the buildings and hang out in the stairway doing whatever.

I remember thinking these girls are crazy for sitting in the park and being felt all up in front of everybody or going in the stairway with someone that you know had just had someone else in there yesterday.

I always told myself "that will never be me." I'll never let a man treat me like that.

Aside from my brother and his friends, all the guys on the block knew there were the girls on the block that all of them could sleep with.

Then to add insult to injury they would brag about it and call them names like hoe, slut and bitch.

When my brothers friends came to our apartment they use to talk about it, laugh about it and compare notes.

You would have thought they were talking about robbing a bank the way they use to talk about getting in and out with quickness.

I swore to myself that would never be me.

I would never even give a guy the opportunity to disrespect me like that.

I wasn't dating or having sex at that time but I was old enough to understand when they were talking about running a train on someone they weren't talking about being a train conductor working for the MTA. Especially when they started mimicking the sounds these girls made and talking about whose vaginas smelt like fish as they were laughing.

These were people I knew. I remember thinking to myself oh my god, suppose that was me some guys were talking about and laughing at. I knew when I started dating I was going to play a whole different ballgame.

I knew I was going to demand respect and have standards.

I also knew, I was going to have to earn it, by not being like one of those many girls you can just take to the staircase.

As I got a little older and started hanging out in the clubs the same clubs me and my girlfriends use to frequent a lot of ballplayers use to hang out at.

One night I met this basketball player from a New York team and he invited me to his car wash.

I didn't understand this invitation. I remember thinking to myself a car wash? What kind of date is a car wash? But at that time I was a little excited to have a date with a professional ball player so I agreed. He gave me the address and that Saturday I went to his car wash.

The first time I met my new friend at his car wash the whole conversation consisted of "what's up" when I first arrived and nothing else until I got up to leave. He then asked me if I could meet him there again. I agreed, I'm not sure why, probably because he was cute and a ballplayer, never the less we set a date and a time then I left.

The second time we met, I had my hopes up for a little more of something this time. A little conversation about me, about him, about anything. I wasn't quite sure what he wanted. I was a little puzzled.

When I arrived, surprise!! He said his favorite two words "what's up." I replied nothing much then sat down.

At least ten minutes went by without anything else being said so I decided I would start a conversation, maybe he didn't know how or was shy I didn't know.

I finally said wow this is a really nice car wash. He in return said thank you would you like me to show you around?

I felt relieved, I remember thinking maybe he just needed a little prompting. Getting a car wash tour wasn't my idea of fun but it was better than sitting down speechless for an hour and glancing at each other every two or three minutes.

As we started walking through the car wash we walked into this room that had a couple of couches a television and some vending machines. This man was sitting down watching television. As my friend and I walked in, he jumped out his seat like he was trying to dodge a bullet and ran out.

I thought to myself O-K maybe he's just trying to give us some privacy. We sat on one of the couches, about ten seconds passed by then boom; Mr. Man of little words turned into an octopus. There were hands all over me.

It was almost like a reaction to an action. The action was we sat on the couch the reaction was his hands all over me.

I had the feeling he'd done this many times before. Maybe this was his game like the guys who took the girls to the stairway; he took the girls to his car wash.

I had to act and act fast. I promised myself I wouldn't be one of those stairway girls and I meant it, so I said the first thing I could think of to get him off of me so I could try and get out of there, I told him I can't, I have my menstrual cycle. It worked he said alright and backed off.

At this point I thought he was a little crazy. The two times I was at his car wash he might have said ten worlds to me and now he expected me to have sex with him, so I played nice because I didn't want to piss him off. I told him I'll come by and see him during the week. I then asked him when he would be around. He told me stop by that Thursday before he leaves town. I said ok and jetted out of there.

Once I got out of there I remember thinking dag he's not only crazy but he's cheap.

This was a million plus basketball player and he either was so cheap or thought I was that he couldn't even spring for a meal before he expected me to open my legs, and at a car wash, what he couldn't afford a hotel?

Had I slept with him in his car wash I would have been like the girls in the stairway not having any standards and therefore not getting any respect?

Love yourself you're a diamond and diamonds don't come cheap.

Needs for Self-Actualization

Everyone needs the basic things in life to survive like food, waters, shelter, air and clothing.

We go to great lengths to keep our bodies' healthy, fit, disease free and safe from danger or harm.

We also go to great lengths to have affectionate loving relationships in our lives and belong to someone or something.

These are all the basic things we've needed since birth.

As we get older, we start to ask ourselves, what do we want to do with our lives? What are our goals? What do we want to accomplish? What do we want to be?

Growing up this was my greatest obstacle in life.

Even though I always loved to write I wasn't that junior high school student who said I'm going to go to college study journalism and write books when I get older, or I'm going to law school and become a lawyer I wasn't sure what I wanted to do so I did everything.

This may not be the traditional way to go about having a career and to some may not be considered normal but if this happens to you just go with it.

The day will come when you will realize your calling and you will aspire to do that which you were meant to do.

We grow up day dreaming our entire lives so don't be afraid to dream.

Dreams do come true I've had many dreams, I've pursued many dreams and have made quite a few of my dreams my realities.

I've owned several businesses, my own home, had a wonderful husband and family and now I'm writing a book. Dreams come true.

Once you realize what it is that you want to do with your life or what your calling is, derive a plan of action to achieve it. Stay focused and don't let anything stop you from reaching your goal.

Give this need the importance of your other needs like getting food and water.

Don't be afraid to aim high. The sky is the limit.

CHAPTER 5

Be Humble

MOVING ON IS going to be a challenging journey. You may need help. Everyone in every walk of life needs help at one time or another. From the time you were a baby you needed help for everything from eating to staying clean.

As you got older you still needed help with getting food, getting clothing, shelter and a place to live. Now that you've grown up, if you're like at least a million other adults you still need help and always will.

No one can do everything that needs to be done in this world by themselves. If you were the president of the United States you would still need help from the Vice President, chief of staff, press secretary, thousands of employees and America just to be voted into office. Let's say you were an artists, be it a singing artist or an actor, you would still need backup singers, a band, or co actors, and camera men. Batman needed Robin and Bonnie needed Clyde.

So it only stands to reason that you need help too. Asking for help may not be the easiest things to do, but remember the very same people you go to for help needs help to for one thing or another.

Don't think asking for help will make you seem weak, incompetent or needy.

I asked some of the most successful people I know who are Doctors, nurses, administrators, professors and business people if they need help and if so how do they ask for it. Their overwhelming response was "of course".

Here are a few of their suggestions:

- When asking for help make a reciprocal offer. For example, if you ask someone to help you find employment, offer to take them out to lunch or dinner once you start working, or if you ask someone to help you find an apartment, offer to cook them dinner once you get moved in.
- Instead of asking someone for what you need, verse it as a favor. You can say something like, I need to ask you to do me a favor, or can I ask you about something I need help with, then tell them why you need help with it.
- Be polite.
- Always be appreciative.
- Always express gratitude.
- Be warm
- Let people do things to help you in their own way.
- Be funny (as possible)
- Try to find someone who identifies with your particular problem. If they've been through it themselves, they'll be more willing to help you, because they can relate to your dilemma.
- Be direct
- Be clear

- Be honest, never try to manipulate someone's help. Your plea will come off as not being genuine.
- Stay positive, believe that people like helping others, which is basically true.
- Try to give advance notice.

Family

Though I believe were all Gods property, God give us parents and family to be guardians over us while were living. He places these people in our lives to care for us, educate us and help us in our time of need and we all have a time of need.

No matter who your family members are whether their biological family members or court appointed family members one of their obligations is to help and care for you. If this isn't possible there are other options, but if your family is in your life they're a great resource to go to for help. Don't be afraid, remember you have to develop courage and face your fears if you're going to move on.

If they love you and can help you more than likely they will.

Make your problem or situation a family problem.

Make your family an active part of the problem and solution by communicating with them about the problem, and letting them help you come up with a solution and resolving it.

When it comes to your family definitely let them help you in their own way.

Your family probably knows you almost as well as you know yourself so they may have a little insight into a way to help you that you may not have thought of yourself.

Their also looking at your situation from another point of view so they probably will have another point of view. They may be able to bring logic to what may be a very emotional situation for you. Don't you know your mother, father, brother, sister, daughter, son or aunt and what they may need, like, or what may make them happy or feel better?

Well they know you too, so they could be most helpful. Be polite and appreciative and ask them for help. Make sure you let them know if they ever need your help you'd be there for them too.

Friends

Most people have either asked a friend or had a friend ask them for a favor before.

If a friend is a true friend they'll care about you and be happy to help you if you ask for help.

If your friend is a fake friend well, you'll probably figure this out as soon as you ask for help, they'll either disappear or like Ike Turner said have more excuses than a person going to jail. Be mindful when asking for help from a friend, reach out only to friends who have proven to be true friends.

Sometimes you can't tell the difference, but be aware that a friend who is not a true friend may take the information you share with them during your time of despair and use it against you for their own personal reasons or gain.

This may only complicate things for you as you attempt to get a handle on your situation.

True Friends

After being in a car accident I had to take public transportation for a while.

A girlfriend of mine that worked at the same company I worked for though it was a different location knew of my situation and offered to take me home every day from work until I got my own ride.

Notice, I said she offered me a ride. A true friend, you may not even need to ask for help. If you're in a spot they'll offer the help to you.

Have you ever offered your assistance to someone in need? You probably did this because you cared enough to want to help them. The same thing stands for a friend who sees you in need. What people do is often more relevant than what they say. Like with anyone else, try to exchange a favor for a favor. This will show your gratitude and appreciation. This will also make it easier for you to ask for help if the need arises again.

Your friend will know your help is appreciated and you're not just looking for a free ride. In exchange for the rides home I offered to put gas in my friend's car for her.

She was doing something for me, and I was doing something for her.

Fake Friends

When I was working at a hospital I was getting to know someone I was interested in. Though this man approached me first, I quickly saw the prospect of us having any kind of relationship was going to be a complicated journey.

At the same hospital I had developed a close friendship with a fellow co-worker. We had similar backgrounds. We were both widowed at a young age and were single moms trying to just make it, so we bonded quickly. We celebrated each other's birthday's together, started hanging out at clubs and burning up the phone all day and all night talking about anything and everything.

I am very private person, but after my girlfriend noticed how friendly me and my gentleman friend were, when we were conversating with each other at the hospital, I confessed to her that me and my new gentleman friend were quickly becoming close friends.

I further explained to her that I had some concerns that he may be playing games and I wasn't sure if I should continue to talk to him. My girlfriend replied by telling me she had seen him around the hospital a longtime and that he was a player and I should leave him alone.

This surprised me because this didn't seem like his character at all. She continued to say everything she could to deter me from pursuing our relationship any more. The following week I was looking through a window at the hospital unit I worked on and noticed my girlfriend standing in the lobby of the first floor by the entrance to the hospital as though she was waiting for someone.

Sure enough my friend walks through the front door. My girlfriend follows behind him and tries to talk to him. He kind of shrudded her off. I didn't think much about it until the following day. My gentleman friend being the creature of habit he was, walked through the front entrance door the same time the following day, and my girlfriend was right there running behind him again trying to talk to him.

The following day she did the same thing again. Each time he shrudded her off, but I realized why she tried to deter me from pursuing a relationship with him, so she could pursue him herself. I was very hurt.

Not only was I faced with the obstacle of whether to continue a relationship with my gentleman friend but now I had an additional obstacle of moving on from what I thought was a true friendship with my girlfriend.

She obviously was using the information I gave her about me having problems with my gentleman friend as an opportunity for herself. Be careful and remember what people do is much more relevant than what they say.

Church

A house of worship is always a good place to go to for help if you belong to one.

Even if you don't belong to one and have nowhere else to turn to, most churches are occupied by god fearing Christians that are dedicating their lives to the lords work. It is very unlikely that anyone in a church would turn you away if you asked them for some form of help, whether its food, clothing or shelter, ask.

If they cannot help you they'll probably guide you to someone or place that can help you. If you don't belong to a church it is a good idea to consider joining one. A church is a good venue to learn about the word of god and worship with other people.

Visit many churches until you find one that is right for you.

If you choose not to go to church pray at home, in your car or at work any time of day or night. Ask god for help with whatever you need. With god in your life all things are possible.

Hospital

If you need help with a medical issue go to the emergency room.

I use to work in the admitting department at the hospital for years. With or without insurance they cannot turn you away.

Work

Different jobs have different benefits. Check with your jobs benefits department to find out what benefit package you're entitled to. I needed assistance with my college tuition so I called the benefits department and found out I was entitled to tuition reimbursement.

This was very beneficial to me throughout my journey of obtaining my education.

The last college I went to was Adelphi University. The tuition there was very high and without some help from different sources I wouldn't have been able to afford the tuition.

School

Most schools, grade school through higher education, have free or discount services for their students. Whatever your need, go to your counselor and find out if your school can assist you.

Schools are a great resource for finding employment. Most schools have a vocational department to help you with everything from getting your working papers to helping you obtain a resume or employing you themselves.

These are services orchestrated for your use. You will find them very useful for those money obstacles we all have at one time or another.

Therapy

Often when faced with crisis and obstacles as you attempt to move on with your life you may become depressed. This is a normal reaction especially considering the circumstances.

It's happened to me as well as millions of others. I once took an abnormal psychology course in which depression was discussed and stated to be normal.

Never being depressed was considered to be abnormal because the majority of people suffer from depression at one point or another in their life. What the majority of people do is what is considered normal behavior.

When you become depressed it is highly recommended to seek therapy upon your onset of symptoms.

The following are some symptoms of depression. Learn to identify them so you can get the help you need. Depression is a mental illness.

Remember if your mind isn't right you won't be able to properly function enough to barely get out of bed much less move on.

Depression Symptoms:

- You may feel sad or down
- You may have trouble eating
- You may have trouble sleeping
- You may sleep a great deal more than usual
- You may feel worthless
- You may feel hopeless

- You may lack energy
- You may feel agitated or jumpy
- You may feel suicidal
- You may act on dangerous impulses
- You may feel panicky
- You may feel delusional

Therapy involves sitting down with a trained professional therapist and talking about your situations, crisis and obstacles using a treatment called cognitive behavior therapy.

This therapy consists of simple techniques which focus on the negative thought patterns which a depressed person usually uses. The therapist will educate you on how depression may be caused by these negative thoughts called cognitive distortions.

Different types of dysfunctional faulty thinking is discussed such as misattribution of blame, assigning blame or thinking things are all or nothing instead of the reality of having options and over generalizing or exaggerating the extent of a situation.

The therapist will encourage you to write down your thoughts throughout the day as they occur so you'll begin to understand how common and often these thoughts are occurring.

The therapists will then begin to discuss these thoughts and behaviors with you that could be associated with feeling depressed. Therapists do not discuss emotions associated with these thoughts and behaviors. Therapists believe that by changing your thoughts and behaviors this will change your emotions.

Much of the thoughts and behavior associated with depression are maladaptive behaviors, which have been learned over a process of time, therefore these behaviors can be unlearned as well. You will be trained in assertiveness, relaxation and desensitization to feared objects.

Remember fear is that obstacle that will cripple you by leaving you anxious and depressed. The manner, in which you view yourself and the environment, will also be examined in order to provide you with the best technique for modifying the maladaptive thoughts and behaviors you may have.

Medication

Along with talking to a therapist you may need some medication to assist you while you're still experiencing mental pain and difficulty coping with problems and obstacles.

Psychotherapeutic medication controls your symptoms of depression. It doesn't cure it.

It's like having a toothache and taking something for pain but you still need to have the tooth taken care of.

Therefore you may need to combine the two treatments therapy and medication to get the results you need. Your health care professional will prescribe the appropriate medication for you.

Prayer

The bible is full of scriptures that can be used as prayers which are perfect for any obstacle, crisis or situation you are going through. As supreme as the bible is, you don't need a bible or a scripture to pray.

You can pray any place in your bed, in your car, in a closet, at one in the morning or three in the afternoon and god will hear you.

Just ask for what you want, what you need and god will be listening. You may not get it when you want, but you will get it, if its gods will and if it's meant to be when the time is right.

CHAPTER 6

Getting Past the Grief

THERE IS NOTHING more traumatic than the death of a loved one. This is probably the most devastating obstacle you will ever need to get past, but you can and will be able to move on with your life in time.

Everyone grieves differently, but once you get through your grieving process you will begin to move on in your journey to recovery. Getting past the grief of losing my husband, brother, and father was the most difficult thing I've ever had to do. Focusing on how they lived, how they loved me, and all the lessons I learned from their love, helped me to get through my grieving process.

As I moved on with my life I kept them in my heart and mind each and every day. The journey I shared with these extraordinary men while they lived set a tone for the journey I would continue on with after their death.

I have a set of standards I live by and love by in part by the things they taught me. Let every life experience you've had with a deceased love one be a life's lesson. Let the time you've spent together have a significant meaning in your life today.

Milton

My dad was the first man I ever loved and respected. He taught me about loving and upholding the responsibility a father has for their child. My mom and dad separated when I was young but we remained close. After the breakup of my parents' marriage my father never missed a weekend of picking me up and spending quality time with me.

We shared a love for music so every headlining act that hit the Apollo we were there. I was probably the best dressed girl in junior high school because every other weekend we went on a shopping spree.

There was never a week that went past that my father didn't have an envelope with some cash in it for me and one for my mom to help us financially. He was still taking care of his responsibility as a father; therefore I grew up believing this is what a man is supposed to do.

As I grew older I knew the man I would have children with would need to be the type of man that would never divorce his children regardless of what happened between us. This is the type of man I wanted. This is the type of man I ended up marrying and having a family with.

Randy

Everything I learned about friendship I learned from my brother. My brother was more than just a big brother he was my best friend.

My brother had his first job as an accountant and left home when I was just sixteen, but a day never went by without us at least talking on the phone for hours like old girlfriends do. If you saw a guy and a girl hanging out in the park in Harlem on a hot summer night that was probably me and my brother. If you saw a guy and a girl on the dance floor of three or four different clubs nearly every Saturday night that was probably me and my brother.

Most importantly if you walked into my hospital room when I was there after having a minor surgery and saw a guy visiting me and bringing some of my favorite things that was my brother. My brother taught me about forgiveness which is very important when it comes to friendship. We never held on to any disagreements we truly moved on from it, buried it in the past, and it was never bought up again.

Like a true friend my brother became my strength when I had no one and accepted my weakness as though they were his own. I was able to talk to my brother about any and everything. Many of my secrets were buried with him.

When I lost my brother, I lost my best friend but I'll never lose the standards I have that he taught me when it comes to having a true friendship.

Steven Sr.

I was relaxing with my friends in Brooklyn when this guy in what looked like army gear walked by me and said hello. My mother taught me to always speak to people when they speak to me so I said hello back no matter how crazy he looked.

It was nearly ninety degrees outside and this guy had on army gear with some heavy black boots. After I said hello back this guy decided to stop and talk to me. OMG was the first thing I remember thinking, I was wondering if the army knew he went A-Wall.

This guy who had to be burning in all that stuff he had on actually turned out to be pretty cool and polite when he started talking to me. He told me his name was Steven and asked me what was my name.

I told him my name and I have to admit I was a little intrigued. This man seemed ok, but looked a little crazy. At that time I liked the excitement of a little crazy. He also sounded intelligent and I definitely liked intelligent. We talked for a little bit then exchanged phone numbers.

This was the beginning of many years of learning how a man should treat a woman when he loves her, and how a woman should be treated by a man. Steven and I started dating. We took it slow, so slow at times I wondered if he was really interested. As time went on I realized this was how it was supposed to be. A man isn't suppose to try and just jump on you if they're really interested. They will invest their time in you and get to know you.

The dates were like nothing I had experienced before. Not only was he investing his time, but he was investing his money in me. We went to nice restaurants, the theater, concerts and sporting events. The holidays started rolling around, my birthday, Christmas and valentine's day. As the holidays came so did the gifts and with each holiday the gifts became more and more elaborate.

I wasn't just opening gifts, but my eyes were becoming opened as well. Men love to give you little tokens of their love and appreciation of you, if they love and appreciate you.

As time went on and the common obstacles that life throws your way started to appear Steven never disappeared, he was always right there. With each year the time, the gifts, the love and support surfaced more and more. Throughout the years Steven's attitude never changed.

We were never faced with episodes of lying and cheating that have become an epidemic in so many relationships. Steven was an un-selfish man. Lying and cheating are selfish acts and true love is anything but selfish. We eventually shared a home and a family together until he passed away.

The Grieving Process

Your life will change when you lose someone that was a significant part of your life. Learning to adapt to change is an obstacle like many others that are full of mental and physical challenges.

Take baby steps one day at a time until you've made it through the grieving process then you will be able to more successfully move on to a new routine. You may experience some or all of the following symptoms which are all normal reactions to grief. You will get through them. They will lessen and eventually disappear with time.

- Confusion
- Numbness
- Emptiness
- Trouble breathing
- Trembling
- Trouble sleeping
- Trouble eating
- Anger
- Guilt
- Nausea

The following are the steps in the grieving process. If you find yourself stuck in a step and don't feel you can make your way past it seek help from either a family member, friend, therapist, church family member, or anyone that you can confide in so you can get past that step and be able to move on with your life.

Denial

- You won't be able to admit to yourself what's going on.
- You'll think you're just going through a rough patch.
- You really don't want to know right now.
- You're to afraid to admit you need a change or to move on so you keep ignoring the situation.
- You'll act as if there is no problem at all, which is a defensive response to protect you from pain, hurt, and suffering.
- You'll start to build up a mask to hide feeling or emotions behind.
- You may experience delusional thinking leading to a feeling that everything is ok when it isn't.
- You may prolong the time before you must confront the pain, hurt, and suffering involved in your loss.

Anger

- You must go through anger if you're going to process your grief.
- You may feel anger at your loved one for leaving you.
- You may be angry at yourself for not being there more, doing more or being more supportive even if you were these things.
- Don't repress the anger
- Acknowledge the anger
- Write in a journal
- Work with a counselor
- Get anger management therapy

Bargaining

- You may begin to make deals or compromises with god or a higher power, for example you may ask to have your loved one brought back and in return you will be the model Christian who is good to everyone and reads the bible everyday or any number of bargains. This is very unlikely to happen. Ask god or your higher power to give you the strength and wisdom to get through your journey and help you to move on instead.

Depression

- You may feel helpless, powerless, and overwhelmed with sadness. Surround yourself with supportive friends and people that you love who will make you feel better.
- Seek professional help depression is a mental illness that may need a combination of clinical therapy and medication to cure.

Acceptance

- Believe it or not you will eventually reach a day when you will accept your loss.
- You will pass back and forth between above stages.
- You will one day find these stages are finally done.
- You will no longer feel angry or sad.
- You will no longer try to negotiate or fix things.

The Break Up

If you've lost someone due to a breakup, change can give birth to a life full of opportunities. You need to open yourself up to these opportunities. Let the person go that you had the break up with.

Don't hold on to anything. Let the relationship end. Don't have any contact at all with this person. Don't focus on any memories. Healing will take place when you learn to forgive and forget.

Forgiving

Your memory may not let you forget, but you can choose to forgive only then will you be able to truly move on. Forgiving is something you do for yourself. When you don't forgive and hold onto the past hurt, your living in the past and not giving yourself a chance to move into your future.

You've loved before and you will love again. If you don't let go of all the anger betrayal of the past, you will not be able to have the loving relationship you deserve in your future.

The last thing you want to do right now is take anger and bitterness into a new relationship. This will probably happen if you carry all the chaos and hurt from your past relationship with you because you haven't been able to let go. Letting go may take you some time. Forgiving will be the first step to letting go, but since your mind might not let you forget you'll need to re-focus your mind in a new direction.

Focus on yourself. You are going to have a little more time for you now. Even if you didn't want to get extra time for yourself this way, turn it into a positive thing and enjoy it. Time is so valuable and it's something we all have to little of. Spend time on your interest, whatever it is your interested in now is the time to pursue it. Whether it's knitting, crocheting, or remodeling your apartment you will now have the time.

Work on a new goal. This is a perfect time to work on some of those dreams you may have. You may want to take a new class and learn something new. There are at least a dozen different classes that meet for about three or four months that teach a lot of very cool topics. It is also a good way to meet new people.

You may want to go all out and work on getting that degree you always wanted. You may want to start a business of your own. A lot of colleges offer a short course on starting your own business or you may choose to start an online business from home.

If you're not already a member of a fitness club now would be the perfect time to focus on getting fit. Exercise is wonderful and necessary for your mind and your body. These are just a few ideas. Come up with an idea of something that will make you happy to do with your free time, as long as your focusing on you.

Losing someone due to a breakup is still a lost so you may have to go through a grieving process. Allow yourself time to grieve if necessary, but try not to focus on the person you've broken up with or the past.

During this period while you're trying to move on be selfish. Focus on yourself, your likes and your interests. As you start to meet new people make choices about people and relationships based on your wants, needs, and standards.

Remember focus on you and make you happy for a change.

CHAPTER 7

Your Self Actualization

EVERYONE IS HERE for a reason. It may take some people ten years to figure out what that reason is. It may take others twenty years, or even a lifetime to figure out their reason for being here. However long it takes, its o-k. Figuring out your purpose in life is the key to your happiness.

No matter how long it takes you, start on your journey, if you haven't already and find yourself actualization. Discover what you should be doing in this life and then continue to move on until you've reached that goal. Then and only then will you be completely happy.

Growing up as a youth, I use to go to church on Sundays and listen to the minister tell the congregation, what's for you is for you. My problem was even though I understood I would be getting out this life what was meant for me to receive, I didn't know what my purpose was, what I should be doing or exactly what I wanted to do, so I tried many things.

The first thing I truly enjoyed doing was writing. I used to sit on my mom's bed when I was thirteen years old and write poetry. My mom was in school working on her master's degree and had numerous papers she had to write. She would often get an A on the papers I helped her with. I even dabbled a little with writing song lyrics, but I never pursued writing, I just continued on with my life like most kids, having fun and not taking anything seriously because that's what kids do.

Somehow between thirteen and seventeen, I decided I wanted to be a lawyer. I'm saying somehow because I have no idea how I came up with this conclusion. Though I find the law fascinating it isn't writing. I decided to apply to John Jay College of criminal justice in New York City and enroll as a pre-law major. I started studying pre-law.

While I was in school studying, I noticed my interest in the law started to diminish. This could be in part due to the lifestyle I was living at the time. I was married, a new mom and had tons of deadlines in school. Don't get me wrong I was happily married and loved being a mother, but I didn't feel complete. Though I was happy with my family I wasn't happy with myself.

The Fight Attendant

As I was looking through the newspaper, I happened to notice the airlines were hiring flight attendants. I remember thinking to myself, what would be more exciting than traveling the world and getting paid to do it. I decided to go to one of the open interviews at one of the airlines that was hiring.

The first interview I went to was nothing like I expected it to be. There had to be at least two hundred applicants lined up around the building. It was like I was auditioning for a reality show. I waited on line for about two hours, and then finally made it to the entrance doors, where the interviewers were anxiously waiting to greet us with coffee, donuts, bagels, water and a smile, so I started smiling as soon as I walked in.

Everyone received a number and a stack of papers to fill out as we sat there for at least another hour before the numbers started being called. I had number 76 and believe it or not it didn't take that long for them to get to my number. I remember thinking we waited for hours and hours to get inside and each interview seemed to last ten minutes tops. What could they possibly find out about a person in ten minutes?

Finally I made it to the interviewer, an immaculately dressed women, attractive with a southern accent and a big smile, held out her hand for me to shake it then sat down and asked me two questions. How would I describe myself and why would I like to be a flight attendant? I answered her questions, then we spent the next five minutes looking over my job application and that was that. I was then told thank you for coming and that they would be in touch. I remember thinking to myself as I walked away I was waiting to be interviewed for nearly three hours from the time I arrived at the hotel the interviews were being held at.

Two weeks later, I received a phone call from the airline. They wanted me to come in for a second interview. I was so happy. I instantly started thinking about all the places in the world I was going to see when I started working as a flight attendant. I didn't get a job yet, but I'm an optimistic person. This is the only way to be.

I had my second interview that following week. The two hundred people that were there three weeks prior were dwindling down to around fifty people. My second interview was much more intense. Instead of one very well put together woman with an accent asking me a couple of questions. I was interviewed by three very well put together women with three different accents, asking me at least six or seven different questions. We even had to watch a film about the airline. Thank god I didn't fall asleep. It was very early in the morning and the film was kind of boring, but I got through it.

Once I left I was feeling pretty good. I had been called for and made it through two interviews for a major airline. I also had met some nice people with whom I had exchanged phone numbers with in the process, now all I had to do was wait and see what happens. Three weeks later I received a phone call welcoming me to the airline and informing me I had to be available to fly to St. Louis Missouri to take my physical as a part of the hiring process.

I was so proud of myself. The competition was pretty stiff. The group of fifty women were all attractive and the ones I had the opportunity to speak to all seemed pretty nice. I was excited and honored.

Around six weeks later after much planning with my husband and making arrangements for my child's care while I was on my journey, I found myself on my way to the airport like a real flight attendant to be.

We were greeted at the gate, escorted on the plane and even introduced to the flight attendants and the pilots. We were VIP's. Once I was escorted to my seat before takeoff as the instructions were being given, the unthinkable and unimaginable happened, I went into a panic attack. I had never been on an airplane before and had no idea I would be afraid of flying. I was like a bride taking several months to plan a wedding and not being able to say I do and finalize the deal because she's too afraid.

I was calmed down by the flight attendants, the plane proceeded to go to St. Louis, I even went through with the physical, but needless to say I didn't get the job. Someone probably made it known what I had just found out myself. I was afraid of flying.

After several months passed by, I started to get over the fact that I wasn't going to see the world, at least not with this airline or as a flight attendant. I started realizing, being a flight attendant wasn't meant to be. It wasn't my calling, it wasn't my destiny. Some things just aren't meant to be.

The Paralegal

I came very close while I was on my journey to become a flight attendant, of making my own money again, it had been a while. As fabulous as my husband was I didn't feel complete just being a housewife, mother and student. These positions are admirable but, I needed more for myself, so I took a short nine month paralegal course.

I knew a little something about the law after studying the law in college for a couple of years, so I didn't think the paralegal course would be to challenging. I believed after completing the course I would be able to get a descent paying job and possibly feel more complete.

I completed the course, received my paralegal certificate and started working as a paralegal part time shortly after. The job I landed paid o-k, but I was stuck in this small law firm pushing papers all day. I stuck it out for a year, but wasn't very happy, so I did what you have to do when your unhappy because life is too short to live unhappily. I moved on.

I started working part for a paralegal firm that had contracts with a lot of different kinds of law firms. The work was more interesting, but I never quite felt like I was where I belonged.

Shortly after I started working at this law firm, the day came that I will never forget, I went to pick up my daughter from pre-school, and believed my daughter was being neglected. I took her out of the pre-school immediately. No one should ever stay in a situation that involves neglect. My daughter comes from my flesh and my blood, therefore neglecting her was like neglecting me, and I love myself to much to be neglected. Moving on was my only option.

Safe Care Child Care

Once I took my daughter out of her preschool I was faced with the obstacle of not having child care for my daughter. Some obstacles will slow down your progress, but they should never stop you.

I looked into a few other pre-schools in the areas in which I lived and worked. I was displeased. This was clearly a problem and like any other obstacle that comes your way, the first thing you should do is to come up with a plan to get past the obstacle so you can continue on with your journey.

CHAPTER 8

Catching Feelings

Being in love is a fabulous addiction. It's a really nice high, unlike anything you'll feel from a drug or alcohol.

On the other hand like a drug addiction that can kill you, the pain of heartbreak can make you wish you were dead. Before getting too involved in a new romantic relationship be clear about who you're getting involved with. Don't make that common mistake most of us women make, don't just look for a male based on attractions like, good looks, perceived intelligence, and financial stability.

Find out what's going on in his head, in his world and in his heart before you give him yours.

Is he interested in being in a committed type of relationship?

- Is he available to be in a committed relationship?
- Is he in healthy relationships with the people in his life?
- What are his views on love, marriage, sex?
- How does he treat people?

The only way to accurately find out this kind of information is to get to know someone. This is why it is vitally important to take the time that is necessary to know a person before you give them your heart. This can save your heart from being broken.

Watch what they do as well as listen to what they say. Let's face it some people lie. Pay close attention to body language. This will help clue you in to some of those little details he may conveniently leave out.

There are a few body postures, gestures and facial expressions that may help you to know what someone is all about.

- Ignoring distractions like the phone or other people shows their interested
- Stillness; when a listener is still this is an indication that their not paying attention to anything except the person their listening to.
- Leaning forward-when you're talking to someone and their leaning slightly forward this indicates their trying to hear everything you have to say.
- Gazing—when a person's looking at you without taking their gaze away they want to hear more.
- Slow nodding-encourages a person to keep talking vs. fast nodding which generally means, hurry up I have other things to do.
- Interest noises-like uh huh means their usually interested in hearing what you have to say.
- Parroting or paraphrasing usually means someone is reflecting your thoughts and understanding what you're saying.

There is also deceptive body language that someone may show when their concerned with not being found out. Their body may show anxiety, send signals of tension and sudden movements like twitching, sweating, minor twitching of muscles around the eyes and mouth and changes in voice tone and speed.

Look for the following anxiety signals.

- Biting of nails.
- Biting of inside mouth
- Patting hair
- Forced smiles-mouth smiles but eyes don't
- Drift off, pause or hesitate as they think about what to say during speech
- Over or under react to things because their natural timing is off.

Once you've given yourself time to find out the type of person you're getting involved with and what their wants and needs are from a romantic relationship with you, then you can feel safer with handing over the part of your body that keeps you alive, your heart.

The relationship I had with my husband who was my first love was the only relationship I ever had that worked out the way a committed romantic relationship should be between a man and a woman.

We dated and took our time getting to know each other. I learned most of what I needed to know about him before we became intimate, specifically and most importantly he was interested in being in a committed relationship.

He was engaged before but the relationship between him and his fiancé didn't work out. He believed in marriage and wanted to find someone that he could have a family with and share the rest of his life with. He was single and was making himself available to put time into having a romantic committed relationship.

He was very close to his family. His mother, who we visited often, lived in Brooklyn New York. He also had aunts and cousins that lived in Queens New York and Bay City Michigan that we visited often as well.

We talked about love, sex and infidelity. We decided infidelity wouldn't be an option, and it wasn't.

My husband was god fearing and tried to treat people according to the teachings in the bible and the way he wanted people to treat him. I believe my relationship with my husband lasted his lifetime because we gave ourselves the opportunity to find out if each other was what we wanted and needed in a romantic relationship and marriage before we got deeply involved.

We knew there was no doubt in our minds that what we would be getting from each other would be what we desired and needed.

The Non-Committal Type

It's very important to find out if someone wants to be in a committed relationship. If someone is not interested in committing themselves to you, you'll have a better chance of hitting the lottery than getting them to change their mind.

Trying to get them to see things your way through any kind of means fair or unfair is like trying to get a bear that sees you as his supper to play nice and give you a friendly bear hug, It's just not happening. He wants a piece of you and that's it.

He may take a while to get you, but once he does he'll take a piece of you and if you're tasty he'll take a few more pieces. If you don't taste good to him he'll spit you out and go find someone else.

Try to avoid this from happening to you. Ask the commitment questions early enough in the relationship before you put your heart into it. There is a chance the truth may not be told. If you have any suspicions or if there's any indication that someone is not interested in being in a committed relationship, read them until you know the truth.

Pay close attention to their actions and give yourself time to read them right. The earlier you move on from a bad relationship the easier it will be for you to do so. It's like catching a disease in its earlier stages you'll have a much better chance of having a full recovery.

I once dated this man that I wasn't really interested in getting into a relationship with because I wasn't looking for one at the time. I kind of went with the flow and didn't ask him the important relationship questions you should ask someone your dating, like his views on commitment, sex, family, marriage, and life in general. We were just hanging out and before I knew it I started having feelings for him.

I knew I was in trouble because I didn't really know anything about this man I was beginning to have feelings for, so I began to become inquisitive and ask questions. Well this didn't sit very well with him. Every time I asked him a relationship type of question it would turn into an argument which slowly started to put distance between us. He started cancelling dates we made to see each other and his phone calls were now coming far and in between.

After much coaxing I finally convinced him to meet me at the park so we could discuss what was going on with us, I wanted to know what was the problem. I was told things were beginning not to work out because I was catching feelings for him.

You could have knocked me over with a feather. I was shocked, all this time I thought that was kind of the idea.

When two people meet and like each other they become friends. If their attracted to each other they will probably start dating. Once dating for a while it is very possible a relationship can formulate and you just might start to have feelings for each other whether it's planned or not.

Well this wasn't his idea at all, and I never bothered to ask so I was screwed. He never wanted a committed relationship and wasn't going to be in a committed relationship so I ended up having to move on with a broken heart that I could have probably prevented, had I only known this truth from the beginning.

Unavailable for a Commitment

There may be a number of reasons a person isn't available to be in a committed relationship. A couple of reasons that affect a substantial amount of people are time and the fact that their already committed to someone else.

Unless you're willing to live your life in love but yet alone and desiring someone that belongs to someone else, availability should be an important factor when choosing a male to be in a romantic relationship with.

Many of those mates that many of us women choose don't usually become financially stable by sitting at home. They're often out and about constantly on the grind.

For these professional or high achievers time is a luxury that they trade in for other luxuries like houses, cars and vacations so just be prepared. It's not that this type of mate won't have the desire to be with you, they probably won't have the time to devote to having a romantic relationship with you because their spending a half to three quarters of a twenty four hour day working to get their mansions, Bentleys and exotic trips.

Keep this in mind when you consider getting involved with this type of mate. I learned the hard way that some people are just unavailable. I use to work at a hospital in Long Island New York on the hospice unit.

One day I was walking down the hall and looked into one of the units. As I was walking by I saw this man standing at the nurses' station with his head down in a book writing. He quickly looked up at me put his head back down then raised his head back up and gave me a second look.

I was smiling to myself and thinking OMG who is that fine man, but I was working so I continued to walk toward my destination. A few days passed by and I was asked to float to another unit to help out.

I was taking a patients temperature and the same man I had seen giving me a couple of glances a few days before walked in the room and softly asked me "what is her temperature."

I almost forgot how to talk. He was now about a foot away from me standing six feet tall about two hundred and fifty pounds and gorgeous. I somehow got out the answer to his question as I was thinking OMG this fine man is a Doctor.

I had only been working for this hospital for a few weeks and have seen some cute doctors but none quite like this. A week went by and I ran into doctor look so good again. This time he said hello with a big smile on his face. I said hello back mirroring his smile and we went our separate ways.

I continued to run into him at least once a week over the next month or so and we exchanged friendly hellos then kept walking. Then one day instead of saying hi, doctor look so good asked me how was I doing?

This was the beginning of us getting to know each other. The conversations got more and more personal. We eventually exchanged phone numbers and started talking to each other outside of work whenever possible.

I'm saying whenever possible because this doctor's available time was as rare as pink diamonds. He had two businesses was affiliated with four hospitals and made rounds at several facilities that catered to his specialty.

At the beginning of our friendship I use to think he was playing with me because he was always so busy. We could barely see each other or talk. His explanations to me about his busy life fell on deaf ears because I didn't want to hear it. In my mind I felt he started this whole thing and kept it going by contacting me on several occasions when I was ready to throw in the towel.

He would also call me on several occasions and leave me a message to give him a call back, but when it came time for us to hang out he was so busy. It took me some time but I finally realized he was very busy.

There were many days I would see him coming into the hospital at 10:00 at night making a pit stop between his private practices and making rounds at other hospitals. I knew his office opened up at 10:00 am so by 10:00 pm he had already put in a twelve hour day and he wasn't finished yet.

I decided if I wanted to be in his life I would have to deal with and accept the fact that he really didn't have any free time and I'd have to see him whenever I could see him.

We continued to see each other when we could and went on a few dates that were amazing. Eventually as time went on he decided he cared about me too much to only be able to give me 1% of him and I agreed I wanted a whole relationship with someone that was available to give me the kind of relationship I believed I deserved so we moved on and parted as friends.

Dating someone married simply isn't right. Nothing good can come out of something bad, no matter how you try to rationalize it. A married man belongs to someone else, so seeing him on borrowed time is like renting someone's house in the Hamptons for the summer.

It's fun but it's only yours for a short time than you have to hand the keys back over to the owner. Married men will tell you everything and anything to get you to believe their cheating on their wives for some rational reason.

It's all lies. If a man can cheat he can lie. When I was at one of my lower points in my life I dated this man that was married because I found him exciting and I wanted and needed some excitement in my life at the time.

I lived to regret it and paid the price because I started catching feelings for him and got my heart broken. When we met he told me he had only married this woman because she trapped him by getting pregnant and he wanted to give his son a family.

I questioned his honesty from the beginning, but as time went on I noticed he spent some late hours with me and holidays with me. There also weren't any typical times he couldn't be reached which you would expect to be the case with most married men, so I thought maybe his reasons for getting married were genuine and he didn't love his wife.

I thought maybe he had genuine feelings for me, so we continued on with our relationship. As a girl growing up in church I learned what's in the dark usually always comes to light. Suddenly little things started creeping out of the dark.

Things he told me about his wife in the past like he wasn't attracted to her and she was a mean Witch started to pop up into our conversations. He developed a sudden case of amnesia. He didn't know what I was talking about and said he had never said these things to me. I tried to blame it on the alcohol, but truth be told maybe he was just lying to me.

We were a little over a year into our relationship, I had caught feelings and now the truth was coming out when I should have learned the truth by asking questions a long time ago. I also started to notice if we were together during the day he started receiving her phone calls and asking me to be quiet when he talked with her on the phone.

Sometimes reality has to slap you in the face before you wake up. I started realizing 50% of marriages end in divorce and the children are still taken care of if that is a priority like it should be, so why was he still married to someone he claims disgusts him? Probably because he wanted to be!

He wanted to have his cake and eat it to. Before I decided to move on I just had a few more questions about his so called shot gun wedding. I wanted to know what were his intentions regarding his family? Was he ever going to move on like millions of people do every day that are in miserable situations?

The answer to this questions was no. A divorce meant losing his house, his dog and everything he worked for, which is the case for most married men. It's usually cheaper for men to keep their wives than to leave them.

It is possible but the chances of you getting a married man to leave their wives are very slim, so this type of unavailable man is almost a guaranteed heartbreak.

Incapable of loving

Some people are incapable of loving others and having a genuine loving relationship because their only capable of loving themselves, therefore if you're hoping for the love and affection you give to be returned it is very unlikely.

These people have a personality disorder called Narcissism, which is causing them to have a narcissistic idea of love. Their loving someone only to be loved back. They have a tendency to emotionally detach themselves from people and feel suffocated by intimacy.

A narcissist that is in a committed relationship of any kind including marriage will react very negatively to perceived restrictions placed on their freedom and are always seeking new thrills and stimulus. As a result they are serial lovers, have countless empty affairs and are usually mentally or physically abusive in their relationship.

Much of this abuse will derive from the fact that narcissist are unwilling to recognize or identify with the feelings of others. Narcissists often believe people live to serve them. In fact they seldom have any regard for other people's feelings at all.

Narcissistic personality disorder is believed to affect less than 1% of the populations and is 3 times more common in men than women but no one clearly knows the number of people with this mental disorder. It is very uncommon and hard to detect. People with narcissistic tendencies rarely ask for help therefore they don't seek treatment and never get cured.

Narcissist believe their O.K. There's something wrong with everyone else. At the same time the signs and symptoms of a person with a narcissistic disorder or tendencies are very clear.

If you're in a romantic relationship whether it's dating or marriage with anyone that has a probability of having this disorder as challenging an obstacle as it may be, attempt to encourage them to seek help or help yourself and move on.

Narcissists usually have some of all of the flowing characteristics:

- Lacks empathy—has no regards for the feelings of others.
- Exploitation of others—uses people to satisfy their need. Different people serve a different purpose for satisfying different needs.
- Sense of Grandiosity—believes their better than other people.
- Thumbs their nose at society and its laws—Doesn't believe the laws that apply to other people apply to them.
- Arrogant—An offensive attitude of one's own superior worth.
- Jealous—Showing envy of other achievements and suspicious of unfaithfulness in relationship even though he/she is probably out there cheating themselves
- Envy—wanting what others have.
- Manipulative—Skilled at influencing or controlling others to their own advantage.
- Expects favored treatment—Believes they are extra special.
- Constant desire for attention.
- Rage in response to criticism—must always be right
- Selfish.
- Ambitious, productive-usually found in positions of power.
- Charming—history shows so were most serial killers.

Unworthy of Your Love

We all have wants, we all have needs. In order for any of us to be happy our basic wants and needs need to be met. Most men take great pride in being a provider and protector for their families.

If you're in a loving romantic relationship with someone and he is not providing you with your wants and needs this is too important and ingredient to be missing if you're going to have a happy healthy relationship. It's as important if not more important than the sex which I'm sure he wouldn't want to go without, so why should you go without your needs being met either.

By the way, you can survive without sex for months but try surviving without food, clothing, shelter or safety for months and see if you still exist. I was watching this movie on television about this woman who was kidnapped. The kidnappers wanted her husband to pay a million dollar ransom to get her back. The husband paid the ransom without hesitation. After his wife returned home they had financial troubles.

The questions came up during an argument regarding money if the husband was upset that he had to pay a million dollars to get his wife back. The husband said no, he would have paid two million if he had to. I thought to myself wow, this man knows his wife's worth. Meanwhile what was going on in my life was very different.

I was dating this international business man for about a year and a half.

This man had two businesses, a house in an affluent area in New York and several luxury cars. Our fist holiday together was my birthday.

On my birthday I had to remind him it was my birthday, which I knew I had mentioned to him was coming up a month previously, but I thought to myself o-k maybe he just forgot we had only been dating for six months at this point so I let it go. The next holiday we were together was Thanksgiving which was at the end of the same month.

We spoke on the phone we exchanged Happy Thanksgivings and that was that.

I thought it would have been nice to spend Thanksgiving together but maybe he wasn't ready for me to meet any of his family and that was fine.

The next holiday we spent together was the following month. It was Christmas.

We had been dating for seven months which isn't a long time but let me remind you this guy is a baller. He had the money, houses, the cars and the clothes and what did I get nothing. I didn't get a card, gloves, a scarf, nada but a Merry Christmas.

At this point I'm starting to think either he's extremely cheap or he just doesn't think much about me. A month and a half later Valentine's Day rolls around.

Guess what I got? The same thing I got for my birthday and Christmas nothing but a phone call. At this point I'm no longer questioning what's wrong with him or is he just cheap? But I'm questioning myself and why I'm still with him.

Let's fast forwards about five months later. I was in a car accident and thank god I came out of it without a scratch but my car wasn't as lucky. I was working two jobs and going to school, there weren't enough hours in the day for public transportation so I needed a car.

I asked my boyfriend and I'm using this term very lightly, to let me use one of his many cars so I could continue to go to work and school. He told me he would get back to me.

Well each time we talked after that, there was one excuse about his cars or money after another. This is when I finally woke up and realized, if he won't be there for me now so I can get to work and have some quality of life, suppose I was sick and needed him or homeless or needed food to eat would he be there for me? It had been a year and a half and this man wasn't doing anything for me and probably had no plans on ever doing anything for me so I erased his number out of my phone, didn't answer or reply to any of his phone calls and moved on. Always remember you can do bad all by yourself! Free yourself of someone that is not making themselves of any real relevance in your life to make room for someone that can help make your world a better place to live.

Real Love

Being able to identify what real love is and isn't, is something that may take a little time. Use your senses. You should feel it and see it. Over the last decade I've learned that when someone has real love for you they will:

- Demonstrate deep affection
- Give you genuine friendship
- Be patient
- Be kind
- Be supportive
- Appreciate you
- Accept you as you are
- Be generous, this will give him joy
- Want to have an intimate and interpersonal sexual relationship with you.
- Protect you
- Love you unconditionally
- Give you a reasonable proportions of time
- Show you he loves you by going the extra mile
- Keep his promises, show up when he says he will and call when he says he will
- Only have eyes for you
- Be interested in your life
- Introduce you to his family

- Introduce you to his friends
- Be forgiving

ON THE OTHER HAND LOVE IS NOT

- Cheating
- Lying
- Envy
- Bitterness
- Abusive
- Selfish
- Conditional
- One sided

CHAPTER 9

Predators

YOU CAN NEVER judge a book by its cover. The ocean on the surface is one of the most beautiful sights god ever created, but what lurks inside of the ocean are deadly and dangerous predators that will rip you in half with one bite. The same thing applies for the woods. Many families choose the woods as a vacation spot to go camping because of its atmosphere of peace, quiet and serenity, but the danger that lurks in the woods are vicious and deadly predators that prey on the small and the weak everyday as a way of life.

Luckily the ocean and the woods have warning signs of the dangers that lurk within these territories. On the other hand it's very unfortunate that once you're outside of nature's danger zones, unless you're at the zoo where you'll need to use your common sense and not stick your finger inside the cages, there are no warning signs of the predators that lurk amongst us every day.

Predators are like wolves in sheep clothing. A lot of predators come in the prettiest packages like that nice little box that says Tiffinay's on it then once you look inside there's the ugliest ring you've ever seen in your life. Don't get it twisted predators are not usually the hobo on the street looking for food in the garbage. A real predator is usually very cleverly disguised as perhaps a business person, a lawyer, a doctor, your boss at work or the handsome well-dressed man you might meet at the deli.

Predators are some evil and dangerous animals whether their wild animal or a mammal. When in predatory mode and the opportunity presents itself anyone can very easily become their prey. Most predators are usually powerful and smart; they arm themselves with a plan and a technique.

The plan is usually attack someone who they don't believe would attack back and the technique is usually always the same each time. Don't think for one minute this technique hasn't been used before. Predators generally don't change. For predators preying on the weak is their lifestyle.

A wild animal's lifestyle consists of going into predatory mode as a means of survival. They find prey to fulfill their need to eat. A mammal or humans lifestyle when going into predatory mode will consist of finding some prey to fulfill their need for sex, money or some form of criminal activity. Wild animals don't have any other way of getting their food so their savage tactics are out of necessity. When you're dealing with a human that's a predator your usually encountering a very sick and twisted individual that doesn't even view you as a person but more like an object or a thing. Often by the time you've realized you're having an encounter with a predator, you've already been preyed upon. It may be too late to have a preventive action but it is never too late to move on. Predators actions are a part of their lifestyle so what happened to you once will happen again unless you move on.

Prey

Your best defense to not becoming prey to a predator is an offense like in basketball you have the defense that stops the players from making baskets, then you have the offense that makes the baskets that gets the point and wins the game. These players that make the points have the skills to get the ball in the hoop. You too have to be skilled about who you're letting into your life. Know as much about the people in your life as possible. Like ball players don't be weak and don't be vulnerable. Predators are always in survivor mode therefore they look for victims who don't appear to serve as a threat.

Remember for predators there's always a technique. They very seldom just jump on you. Whether it's a wild animal or a mammal there's usually a method to their madness. Get to know everyone you let in your lives. The more you know a person the less likely you will fall prey to any of their foul play.

Technique of Predators

Most predators whether it's a wild animal or a mammal will stalk you until the opportunity arrives for them to attack. They may either watch you for a period of time or get to know you for a period of time until the opportunity presents itself for the kill. As someone's watching and getting to know you. You watch and get to know them. There's no such thing as a stupid questions, so ask plenty of them.

A cougar also known as a mountain lion when in predatory mode usually keeps himself out of site until he sets his eyes on his prey, which is usually some one that is much smaller than him like a rabbit or a small child. The cougar then attacks his prey on the back of the neck. The cougar never attacks any other part of the body like the arm or the stomach but always the back of the neck. This is his technique.

Move On

Male Predators

Warning, many men often view women as prey. Men are very competitive and they love sports. Their sport of choice when it comes to the opposite sex is often hunting and fishing. Like the animals of the wild they also have a type of prey they desire.

This varies, it could be someone who's a brunette, a blond, someone young, someone shapely, someone thin, someone tall, someone short, someone older, someone black, someone white, someone Hispanic, the list goes on and on, but it's usually always someone they don't find threatening like the cougar prefers a heir a much smaller non-threatening animal than himself.

There's also usually a technique as in hunting. They may take their time checking you out by watching you closely then when the time is right like a wild animal go for the kill by taking a big chunk out of your heart.

A predator may use the fishing technique and dangle some bait is front of you like their cars, clothes or money. They'll dangle something attractive enough to make you go for the bait then they'll snatch you up like a fisherman dangles worm as bait to catch fish.

There's almost always a hunting ground. Sharks have the ocean, cougars have the woods and most men believe this is a man's world therefore any place is fair game for them to hunt. Especially places in which they feel territorial over, like a job in which there in a managerial position, their home, their favorite bar, club or their neighborhood.

The hunting ground of an animal and mammal is not the same, but the end result is very similar pain and destruction. The only substantial

117

difference between the journeys of an animal versus a man when in predatory mode is the destination.

Animals go on a journey to capture their prey as a means to survive. They need to eat. There's no one in the ocean or the woods cooking these animals some fried chicken, oxtails, macaroni and cheese and greens, so they have to get their meals the only way they know how and that's by hunting their prey then killing them for a meal.

A man's journey when hunting their prey is usually to satisfy a need for sex. They always look for someone unthreatening to make this journey as easy and quick as possible.

Once he gets what he was looking for he'll have reached his destination. It's sad but very simple. Men, who are looking for an easy lay, go after the easy prey. These men are looking for women who will give them what they want easily and won't pose too much of a challenge. They enjoy that thrill of the hunt. Often these men are looking for the women you'll find at a club who will sleep with a man after being served one or two drinks, or will sleep with a man on the first date or in some cases no date at all.

I've had men come up to me at a club and ask me to do them a favor to help them out with their itch. Since when is having sex with someone a favor? They can scratch themselves they have two hands. When men are eyeing you as an easy prey don't make yourself so easy to catch. This is why their picking you because your easy and gullible.

Like the cougar in the wilderness that pounces on the heir, an easy target instead of another cougar, a wolf or a bear that would be much more challenging and fulfilling.

They want a quick meal and the heir is easy. The wolf or the bear would put up a fight that perhaps couldn't be won.

If the cougar was looking for someone to mate, you could bet your last dollar he would probably look for another cougar or a more challenging animal. He just wants the heir for an easy quick meal, just like the man who wants unchallenging women for some quick sex.

It's a quick journey to a quick destination than it's on to the next one.

Throwback

A man when fishing will sit in wait for hours patiently to catch a fish. Those fish that bite in the first few minutes usually get thrown back and the wait continues for that fish that isn't so easy to catch. It's this fish that is always so much more appreciated because they were made to wait for the catch.

Don't allow yourself to be an easy prey. Aren't you a good catch? Aren't you worth waiting for?

Unlike those poor heirs or unfortunate small fish or swimmers in the ocean you can better control your fate of becoming someone's prey for the purpose of sex. When you meet someone if there's an interest and an attraction you can set the tone and turn a predator-prey situation into a friendship or a possible loving romance that could possibly turn into wedding bliss.

You will be preyed on by men so make it what you want it to be.

He'll have an agenda so let him know what your agenda is. Keep it 100% real from the beginning. If you're looking for friendship let that be known. If you're looking for a relationship let that be known.

If he's looking for something more than to just to pounce on you and get a piece of you, he'll be willing to wait just like he will for that fish that will take him eight hours to catch, then he'll brag about it for eight months and even hang it over his mantel place to remind him of his great catch for the next ten years.

The same thing applies when it comes to a relationship. If a man has to wait for you, by romancing you, taking you out and getting to know you for a reasonable amount of time, I would suggest at least a few months before earning the privilege of having sex with you; he will more likely appreciate the great catch he's made in catching you for the rest of his life.

8-2-4

I once worked at a job where the position was so disrespected there wasn't even a name for the position, it was given a number 8-2-4 like being in prison you were no longer Mary, mark, Dr. or cashier you were simply known as 8-2-4

While at this job I experienced the worst case of a predatory—prey, relationship imaginable. I equate it to being in prison not only because I wasn't given a title only numbers but I didn't have any rights because I was always wrong. This was the way my supervisors saw it. Someone had to take the blame for all the inadequacies performed as a whole by everyone involved including themselves and guess what I was the unlucky scapegoat all of the time. Like in prison your never right, you're always wrong therefore no matter what goes wrong behind those prison walls if you were anywhere around you will always have to pay a consequence for whatever goes wrong.

In addition to not having any rights, the pay for the job I was doing was much lower than it should have been. I was being paid prisoners wages. My pay was much like prisoners getting paid fifty cents an hour to work heavy machinery. This kind of work would very easily pay upwards of twenty dollars an hour outside of the prison walls. Working this job for two years was like doing two years hard time in a maximum security prison.

Most wardens don't particularly care for the prisoners in prison, which is understandable under the circumstances. Not too many people are fond of murderers, rapist and bank robbers. I found myself in the same situation. My supervisors weren't fond of me though I never understood why. I never committed any crimes unless coming to work all the time on time, being polite, working as hard as my mind and body would allow me to work and trying to be friendly to everyone was a crime. I always thought I wasn't liked just for being me, like the woman who gets arrested because perhaps she looks a certain way or for no other reason than being who she is.

I could make assumptions about why I was made the scapegoat at my job from here until eternity, but at the end of the day I was made to serve hard time for a crime I never committed. This remained true up until the day I left and happened to see a note on one of the supervisor's mailboxes telling her to put in her notes the 8-2-4 failed to do something. By saying this it would prevent them from getting a citation. The truth was there was no truth to this note but the 8-2-4 had 5 hours left at this position and really didn't give a damn.

If you find yourself in a situation like this one and you get the chance to get out of prison leave and make sure you never return. If by some chance lightning strikes you twice or even three times, you keep moving on as many times as you have to until you get it right.

Remember everyone has rights. Exercise those rights. Refer to your employee handbook or a lawyer if you need to. If you're working somewhere where your rights aren't being exercised, you don't need to be working there.

Child Predators

Were still trying to protect our children from what's lurking on the internet.

Internet predators are now stepping out of the screen. They've reached an all-time low. These perverts are now entering our homes.

Like the predators of the oceans or the wilderness they also have a technique, but like the predators at the workplace there may be no initial warning signs. These men are usually very charming ordinary people who seek out single mothers with small children and no man in their lives, or anyone who would pose as a threat.

They romance these mothers and when they believe they've gained their trust and all guards are down they go in for the attack of their young children. This technique is usually very well planned out which is why many of these type of predators are successful in capturing their prey. These women never know what hits them until it's too late.

When small children are involved, you should always have a warning sign attached to anyone knew who enters into their lives. At the first sign of danger, move on before it's too late.

I once dated this man who was very handsome, charming and intelligent. He was everything any women would want in a man. We met, became friends and started dating.

We went to three star restaurants, concerts, museums, movies, plays and always had the best seats in the house. Whenever I was with him, he made me feel like I was the only person in the room.

He was into fitness and introduced me to staying fit by exercising regularly.

He enjoyed tennis so we played a lot of tennis at $200 a game an hour. Money was never an object. We went shopping all of the time. Whatever I wanted I got. My friend enjoyed it when I tried on the clothes in the store before buying them and gave him a little fashion show. It was really cute and turned him on. This was his little reward for spending obscene amounts of money on me in these stores. Before leaving the store we always made a pit stop to the perfume counter to purchase the expensive perfumes I loved so much because he loved the way I smelled and I love to smell good.

Every morning I always received a call saying good morning and at least one call during the day just to see how my day was going. Needless to say I was really falling for this man.

One day I finally asked him "how can it be that you're single" he told me he just never found the right women to marry. We took the conversation a little further by talking about his kids and their mothers. He said he misses his boys since their mothers moved out of New York he rarely gets to see him.

The day we had this conversations is the day all kinds of red lights started flashing. I couldn't understand why not just one woman but two women would move half way around the world and take their children away from a good man that wants to be a father to his children.

As time went on and I sporadically asked questions about his children, their mothers and his relationship with these children it started to become apparent to me that these women weren't just trying to get away from him as I had originally thought, they were trying to get their children away from him as well.

During conversations with a little prompting he started telling me details about his children's mothers' suspicions of him when left alone with his sons and some of the allegations that were made about abuse.

After much prompting he told me he was accused of touching his sons, but listening to him my gut was telling me this was an underline reason why his sons were taken half way around the world.

I knew if this was true he would never admit it because predators are always in survivor mode and will protect themselves at any cost. I became very suspicious of him from this point on. We continued to date, but I never let my guard down. I knew sooner or later the truth would come out.

One night I didn't receive a phone call so I decided to call instead to say goodnight and to my surprise my boyfriend had company. It wasn't one of his men friends or even a woman friend it was his child hood friend's daughter. As I remember the story he told me went something like this.

A friend that he grew up with husband had died and he was helping her with her daughter because she was now alone. My heart dropped this sounded like me. I thought to myself ok when I called and asked him what he was doing he didn't try to hide the fact his friends daughter was there, so there probably was nothing wrong going on.

We talked further and I asked him how old was she, thinking it was a small child or a toddler he said sixteen. I think I blacked out for a minute then I asked him what was she doing playing video games or something he said no she's taking a bath. O-k I heard enough!

Why in god's name would some woman leave her sixteen year old daughter at the home of a forty year old man alone? She was too young to just be a friend of his hanging out and too old to need a baby sitter what was going on?

My mind was racing, before I said something I would regret I thought it was best for me to get off the phone, so I told him I had to get up really early and was tired so I would talk to him tomorrow.

As time passed on my boyfriend was spending more and more time with this sixteen year old girl and spending loads of cash on her. I was very confused because he wasn't hiding it from me but why was he doing it. I started thinking maybe he had adopted her as a daughter or just missed his children or was just trying to sincerely help someone out, it just all seemed really suspect and creepy. I decided I would become a part of their lives then I could find out for myself what was going on.

Each time the three of us planned on getting together miraculously something would come up. My suspicions started to escalate and I started asking more questions.

One of the questions I asked was how did this girl look. His description was startling.

I expected him to describe her by height, weight, race and personality or at least something along those lines, but instead the description went something like "these young girls today are born nice and ripe; all that ripeness must be for something."

I was speechless.

My suspicions continued to grow until one day he called me on my cell I didn't answer so he called my home phone and my daughter answered. He stayed on the phone with her for about twenty minutes asking her personal questions about herself. When I walked in the room I initially thought she was talking to her grandmother or someone she knew. When I found out who she was talking to I flipped.

After this event there was a two month period we didn't speak. I reconsidered and decided to talk to him again. During the first conversation we had he went straight for the kill and had the audacity to ask me how my daughter was and expressed how much he wanted to meet her. My response was, click then a dial tone. I moved on and never answered his phone calls or spoke to him again.

CHAPTER 10

Make a Plan

Being spontaneous is cool. When it comes to going to the mall with your girls or getting some fast food instead of cooking, but when it comes to decisions that mold out your destiny you need a plan. Making a major move in your life without a plan is like jumping out a plane without a parachute, its suicide.

It's very unlikely that you're going to have a successful jump and land on your feet. Plans are made with the intentions of guiding you through and carrying out some kind of action to help ensure your success.

With every plan ask yourself these questions:

- What—what is it that you want to do
- Why—why do you want to take this form of action
- How—how would you like to go about performing this action
- Who—who will be the major players that you will need to be involved with in this action
- Where—where will this action take place

- When—when will this action take place
- Results—what results would you like to see? What is your desired outcome

Then implement the plan and make it happen. Please trust me when I say it doesn't matter what you would like to do, whether its move on from a relationship, a job, or an old life and into a new one. Without planning on having a parachute to land on your feet after jumping out into a new venture you'll splat all over the ground like a pie in a clowns face.

A plan isn't difficult at all. This will be the easiest part of your challenge of moving on. It's never a good idea to merely visualize a plan. You should write it down.

Think about some of the plans we all hear about or plan like a thanksgiving dinner, a vacation or something more challenging like planning a wedding. How disastrous these could turn out if we just went to the supermarket grabbed a bunch of food and drinks then went home, and tried to just cook what we grabbed.

I know for certain I would end up running back and forth ten times because I forgot the simplest things like milk or butter. By the time I finished cooking I would be too tired to eat and would just want to sleep.

Imagine going on a trip without any planning. You may have the what, the why, and the desired outcome covered, but how are you going to get there unless you're going to just get in a car and drive until you get too tired to drive anymore, and that's where you'll have your vacation.

Who's going with you? Without any kind of planning you'll find yourself going on a trip by yourself. Not too many people can just pick up and leave their lives behind to go on a vacation. Where you're going will be a mystery even to you, if you don't have a plan.

Even if you don't have a destination in mind, you have to at least plan a direction. Are you going north, south, east, or west. If you don't at least plan this you might end up going around in a circle. When you're going, I'm guessing without a plan will be never.

Just try to make sure whenever the mood hits you to go on this unplanned trip you at least have the money to get you wherever you're going, and money to eat and have somewhere to sleep when you get there, or else you may starve and have to sleep on the street.

A wedding without a plan isn't going to be a wedding. You may have the covered, you want to get married. The why maybe covered, because you love each other hopefully? The results may be clear what you would like the outcome to be, a happily ever after, but what about how, who, where, when, and implementing your wedding/marriage to make it happen.

How are you going to get married? You can't marry yourself. Who will marry you? Even if you don't make plans with a minister, priest, Rabi, or some man/woman of the cloth in a formal wedding setting you still need someone to marry you.

It even takes some thought of an action to go to a justice of the peace. Where will you get married? At home, in a church, in your backyard? Even if you wake up one morning and say "let's get married today", you still need to have a plan as to where it's going to be and have someone who's qualified come and perform the ceremony for you.

When is this wedding going to take place? In two hours, the next day, next month, or next year. Even if you're ordering a pizza they give you a time table as to when it will be delivered. As you can see without covering some of these important basics this wedding will never happen.

It's like waking up in the morning at 5:00 AM for work without an alarm clock. You're leaving it to chance that you'll wake up. Planning also allows you to take a little time and think about what you're doing before you do it. This can help you to avoid those spur of the moment mistakes that can be a result of spontaneity.

Some mistakes you can recover from, like getting upset with that boyfriend that still has a little promise. Telling him it's over than changing your mind and the two of you decide to work on your relationship.

Some spontaneous reactions you can't recover from so easily, like quitting a job because something angers you at the moment. I have a girlfriend who was upset with her supervisor over her tone of voice. My girlfriend was so upset she not only quit, but she spelled it out to make sure it was perfectly clear. She told her supervisor "I quit, Q.U.I.T. quit!" and walked out.

She went home slept on it then woke up the next day and was without a job. She regretted quitting and said she was just upset, but it was too late. Instead of quitting in the manner that she did, she should have planned to move on by looking for another job, until she found one then give in her job resignation letter or at least two weeks' notice.

It took my friend four months to find another job. Planning gives you among other things the time you may need to make certain your move isn't just a smooth move, but the correct move.

Let's say you move on from a long term marriage or relationship, the time it will take you to properly prepare by finding a new place to live or him finding a new place to live, and make whatever changes or division of assets that will be necessary, will be time to think and be 100% sure your making the right decision and move on.

Moving on is meant to compliment your life and make it better, not complicate it and make it worse. Unfortunately not everyone will be in a situation where you have the option of planning.

Some situations maybe so tragic you'll find yourself in a point of no return, scenario where you'll have to disappear into the dark of night. For those of us that do have the opportunity to plan, a well thought out plan can help us escape from some of the most miserable of circumstances.

If a person can plan and execute an escape from a maximum security prison which is their hell, you can escape from yours. And you don't have to cut through prison bars to do so. When planning always have a plan A and a plan B.

If your initial plan doesn't work out you'll have a second plan to fall back on so you can continue on with your journey.

Ten years ago I decided I wanted to start a business so I drew up a plan.

The plan

- What—a childcare program for children ages 6months to 12 years of age.
- Why—I wanted to establish a place for children to gather while their parents were at work. Where they would be safe, that was affordable, and where they could learn and have fun at the same time.
- How—I needed to find a school where I could get the training I needed to care for school aged children. I found a certification program at York College in Queens, New York so I registered and took the course. Fortunately the program I went to covered children from infants through twelve years of age. Once I finished with the program I decided to take care of children at home, to get my feet wet before opening up an afterschool program. First thing, I did was think of a name that would fit what i wanted to accomplish. I was interested in having a safe place to care for children so i thought of the name safe care. I went and registered my business as safe care childcare. I then started to solicitate business. I made flyers and put them all throughout the neighborhood. In laundromats, restaurant, windshield wipers, every place and anyplace I walked by where there was an opportunity for a flyer. As I waited for people to call me I made my home more children friendly. I bought toys, children books, and children educational videos. I prepared my home to welcome children. I had my first client in about a month; second one about two weeks after that, my third and

fourth one within the following month. I took care of these children for a year in my home. After that initial year, I decided to take my business outside of my home and into a school setting. I started investigated locations. I started going to several business arenas in the neighborhood to find out where there was a need for my services.

- Where—as I was looking for my locations I had an epiphany. I realized there was no better place to have a childcare service for school age children up to age twelve than a school, so I decided to focus on schools as a location for my business. I started going to all the elementary schools in the area and made inquiries on who could help me with my business venture.

- Who—I was directed to seek out the principals of all the schools I was interested in being a location, so that's what I did. I came upon this one school that I was close to where i was living at the time. He thought my vision was a good one, but needed me to write a business proposal so he could give it to all the necessary players. I wrote my proposal. The principal shortly got back to me and told me all the systems were go, I just needed to get permission from the fire and police departments to keep the school building open pass its normal time of four o-clock. I went to the police and fire departments in this neighborhood, showed them my business license and filled out all the necessary paper work. Within a matter of weeks i had the permission I needed to keep the school building opened pass 4:00, for the purpose of having my afterschool program providing I had security for the hours I would be open. I needed security and staff so I started inquiring around the school who would be interested in working at an afterschool program. I started interviewing all the interested parties and hired the staff I would need. I then started making contact with all the city and state agencies to arrange payment to be made to me for all the qualified applicants. I then contacted all of the teachers in the school and made them aware of my business that was opening up as a service to their students, and gave them flyers to distribute to the parents of their students. I then arrange dates for registration of students to the afterschool program.

- When—my afterschool program would be open Monday through Friday from 3:00 pm to 6:00 pm. I would have extended days when the school would have a half a day. On those days I would be open for operation for 12:00 pm to 6:00 pm. My business would operate according to the school schedule. When school was in session I would be open. When the school was closed i would be closed during the school year. During the summer I would have a four week summer session in which my business would be open from 7:00 am to 6:00 pm.
- Results—the results I wanted was to have a successful childcare service that was a safe place of learning for children. I also wanted to make money.
- I implemented my plan. After I went through all of these steps I opened up safe care childcare that September. I had no business experience before i started safe care childcare. I an idea and a plan. Safe care childcare stayed open for six years.

I have spent most of my life in school. Each and every time I went to school I had to plan for it. I would have never been able to start or complete any form of education without having a plan. This plan was a great deal, simpler then starting a business.

A plan doesn't need to be complicated, in fact make it as simple as possible, with the intent on fitting whatever goal you have and making the transition and implementation of that goal as smooth and easy as possible.

The Plan

- What—I wanted to go to school
- Why—to receive a degree to qualify me for a certain profession, to learn a trade to acquire a certain job
- How—I researched several schools that majored or specialized in my field of interest. I then contacted schools I was interested in and requested an application. I completed the applications, paid the fees and took whatever tests or wrote whatever papers were required for each school. I then looked into financial aid, grants, tuition assistance, and tuition reimbursement programs to finance my education.
- Who I contacted the admissions office regarding my application. A guidance counselor regarding my courses and the financial aid office regarding financing my education.
- Where—I wanted to attend schools that were assessable to me and wouldn't cause too much of a hardship for me to commute back and forth.
- When—I needed to find time in my schedule to attend classes. I also considered attending schools that would accommodate my schedule. For instance one of the universities I went to had blended courses as a big part of their curriculum. A blended class will allow you to go to class one half of the time and attend class online the other half of the time, so you can complete your studies more or less at your convenience.
- Results—the results I was seeking a degree or certificate.

I implemented this plan by going to these schools and receiving a degree or a certificate as planned. I once lived in an apartment so terrible that at times when you flushed the toilet the items in the toilet would come out into the shower. I had to move and move fast. As I was constantly struggling with the landlord to fix the plumbing along with numerous other problems in this apartment, I also came up with a plan on how I could move away.

The plan

- What—I wanted to move
- Why—I was living in less than humane living conditions
- How—I started looking for apartments in the newspaper, on the internet, and went to see real-estate agents. I started saving money to prepare for the move. I looked for the most affordable moving company I could find. I started packing up my possessions as soon as I planned on moving to prevent myself from becoming to overwhelmed.
- Who—I started making appointments with the apartment owners and real-estate agents to see all the available apartments that I was interested in. once I found an apartment I also contacted the post office and all the businesses I had interaction with like my bank, job etc. regarding my address change.
- Where—I looked for apartments in areas I liked. In areas that were affordable, that I thought was safe, and that wasn't too far from my place of employment. I also took into consideration certain conveniences like transportation and availability to stores.
- When—I had a very busy schedule, but this was very important so I found time after work, on days off, and when I didn't have to attend any classes.
- Results—I found an apartment that fit the criteria I was looking for

I implemented my plan by moving as soon as I finished all the steps in my plan. Not all plans will be a plan where you'll have to hide money in your toilet tank and hope it doesn't get flushed or underneath the carpet and hope no one finds it and spends it, on a case of forties or a stripper at the club, until you can make your escape in the middle of the night by swimming by swimming across the east river.

Listen you do what you have to do in order to survive and be able to live and laugh again. Some plans are happy ones with a real result. A good plan produces good results.

No matter how big or small whether it's a happy occasion or a sad one, making a plan is like planning your destiny. Your saying what you want to happen, how, when, where, and what you want to happen as a result of your efforts, then you turn around and make it happen.

Remember always document the action you want to take. You don't have to write it in blood. Leave room for change, flexibility, and the what if's, but write it down. Some of the most important courses in history started with the strike of a pen on a course of action that was to be taken, like the declaration of independence, which was a plan to free slaves. One of the most thought out and most rewarding plan was when I planned my wedding.

The plan

- What—I wanted to get married
- Why—because I wanted to spend the rest of my life with the man of my dreams
- How—instead of what some couples traditionally do and go to the bride's family and finance the wedding, we was going to finance it ourselves. Before I contacted anyone I wrote every plan of my wedding down to ensure it was executed exactly the way I wanted it
- Who—I didn't have a wedding planner, we did everything along with the help of a few family members and friends. We first contacted my fiancés minister to get a commitment from him to marry us. We sent out wedding invitations to all of our families and friends. He started contacting different DJ's and bands to supply us with music. We shopped around for florist. We went to some of our favorite bakeries to find the perfect one to make our wedding cake. I shopped around for bridal boutique, and a wedding dress than had my maid of honor and bride's maids fitted for their gowns. I reached out to family members to cook the dishes I wanted according to a menu I constructed. I shopped around for a shoe store that would dye my maid of honor and bride's maid shoes to match their gowns. I found a photographer; I shopped around for bridesmaids gifts.

- Where—we wanted to get married in my fiancés church, so we booked a day to get married. We shopped around for a reception hall to have our reception in
- When—we set the date for the following year in January
- Results—we wanted to live happily ever after

Our wedding plans were implemented beautifully. We got married on January 19th and lived happily until his death.

CHAPTER 11

Re-invent yourself

In my opinion the butterfly is one of the most beautiful creatures on earth. This multi-color beauty doesn't start off fluttering its beautiful wings; it has to re-invent itself from a cocoon to a caterpillar to something so magnificent you can't help but to marvel at its beauty.

Like a butterfly that starts its life as something that's not fully developed then evolves into the beauty it is meant to be, spreads its wings then flies. We too can re-invent ourselves, break out of our cocoons then spread our wings and fly.

What do you want to do, who do you want to be, what destines would you like to reach because the sky is the limit. Every day in every way people are re-inventing themselves and evolving into the people they desire to be and were meant to be. Things like the seasons changing and you're getting older with each change of the season are a change that is inevitable, but some changes can be made by design.

No matter how you slice it you're not going to stay the same. So before your hair is all gray and your teeth all fall out make the changes in your life to make your life the most beautiful and fulfilling life it can be.

Start off with who you want to be. Let's say you're born Lisa McDonald child of Tina and Peter McDonald. When you start school your now Lisa McDonald student. You decide you want to go to medical school, you then become Lisa McDonald M.D. you've just re-invented yourself by your design.

Your friend you went to high school with, who you knew as Tracey Burger grew up and met the love of her life Bruce Washington. Tracey and Bruce got married and Tracey Burger is now Tracey Washington. Tracey and Bruce have a child, now Tracey is a mother. Tracey's daughter gets older and starts grade school, and Tracey joins her daughters PTA and becomes the president.

Tracey has re-invented herself from Tracey Burger to Tracey Washington wife, to Tracey Washington wife and mother, to Tracey Washington wife, mother, and PTA president.

Not all reinventions are strictly by design, but are necessary due to some of those obstacles we come across during our journey in life. We've all known that girlfriend that was first known as Kevin's girlfriend, then was known as jimmy's girlfriend, then became mikes fiancé, now she's Gregory's wife.

You see re-inventing yourself also involves finding the best fit for you, doing what's best for you, and being your personal best. Being your personal best usually involves more than merely changing your name from miss to Mrs. or miss to M.D.

Being your personal best often means re-inventing the way you think, look, act, and view the world. By developing necessary life skills you need like, self-love, courage, knowledge, self-actualization, strength, and being humble so you can go from point A where you're at today to point B where you would like to be, which will ultimately bring you that happiness that you've always dreamed of.

I am living my dreams by going from point A to point B and so can you. Start today, stay positive and never give up. You will have all that you've ever dreamed of and more.